FOURTEEN DAYS ✚O AMAZING HEALTH

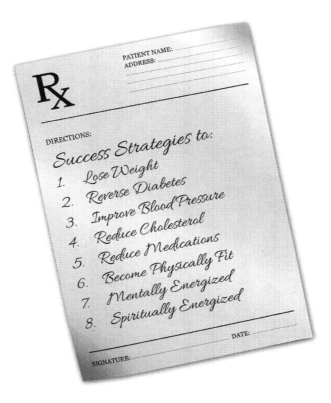

Patient Name:
Address:

Rx

Directions: Success Strategies to:
1. Lose Weight
2. Reverse Diabetes
3. Improve Blood Pressure
4. Reduce Cholesterol
5. Reduce Medications
6. Become Physically Fit
7. Mentally Energized
8. Spiritually Energized

Date:

Signature:

Dona Cooper-Dockery, MD

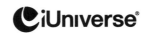

FOURTEEN DAYS TO AMAZING HEALTH
SUCCESS STRATEGIES TO LOSE WEIGHT, REVERSE DIABETES, IMPROVE BLOOD PRESSURE, REDUCE CHOLESTEROL, REDUCE MEDICATIONS, AND BECOME PHYSICALLY FIT AND MENTALLY ENERGIZED AND SPIRITUALLY ENERGIZED

iUniverse books may be ordered through booksellers or by contacting:

iUniverse
1663 Liberty Drive
Bloomington, IN 47403
www.iuniverse.com
1-800-Authors (1-800-288-4677)

ISBN: 978-1-5320-1087-3 (sc)
ISBN: 978-1-5320-1089-7 (hc)
ISBN: 978-1-5320-1088-0 (e)

Library of Congress Control Number: 2016920246

Print information available on the last page.

iUniverse rev. date: 03/25/2017

Medical Disclaimer

This book is intended to educate, inspire, and empower you to make lifestyle changes that will propel you to a healthier, happier, and more fulfilled life. You should use the information received in this book wisely. Always consult with your primary health care provider if you have questions or concerns. The information presented in this book should be used to supplement, not replace, medical advice from your primary health care provider.

To all my patients who have had life-changing experiences using this program—and to you. It is my desire that you too will be inspired and empowered to embrace a healthier lifestyle that will propel you on your journey to a longer, healthier, happier, and more abundant life.

CONTENTS

Part 4: Eat to Beat and Treat

A Doctor's Paradigm Shift

---

*T*he poll numbers are out. My city made breaking news! The McAllen metropolitan area ranked as America's *fattest*. This was in 2012. We held on to that position for two consecutive years and are now in second place. Wow! Just under 40 percent of the people living in the McAllen area, my hometown, are obese. What a position to hold! You will agree with me that this is not a statistic to be proud of but one to cause concern. With this high incidence of obesity come the dreaded diabetes, hypertension, cardiovascular disease, and even early death.

The unfavorable obesity statistic of McAllen, Texas, was my reality a few years ago. The surge in the incidence of poor health is not only a local problem. Throughout the world today, so many people, young and old, are experiencing very poor health. There is an alarming number of people with chronic disease who are dying daily despite the advancement of medicine in this modern era. What, then, is the real problem behind this epidemic of chronic disease and death? Surely there must be a cause. There must be a reason for this gigantic problem that plagues not only the United States of America but many other countries in the world.

As a responsible physician facing this startling reality, I decided to take action and thus become more effective in changing my patients' health care outcomes. During medical school and residency training, the emphasis is on carefully diagnosing and treating diseases, while minimal attention is given to treating the root causes or preventing chronic illnesses. For more than twenty years of my internal medicine practice, I have been faithfully practicing this type of medicine. While I have become very successful, with a very large practice including offices in different cities, there was something missing, something very important, and that was sharing the success strategies for health and longevity with my patients. I needed a paradigm shift in the way I approached health and wellness. The emphasis must be on empowering my patients to take control and make changes that will change lives for the better and positively impact their health destinies. I wanted to influence miracles as patients changed their lifestyles and improve and reverse chronic diseases.

As a practicing physician, I have treated thousands of patients with various illnesses. While I take pleasure in my work, it saddens me to diagnose young patients with diseases that used to be predominantly present in the older and geriatric age groups. Diseases such as type 2 diabetes, hypertension, and coronary artery disease were once known as diseases for the older folks but are now seen in younger populations. This is frightening. You would think that in this modern age and with the advancement of medicine, diseases such as diabetes, heart disease, and cancer would be eradicated, as were smallpox and polio. However, sadly, the reverse is happening. Patients continue to develop complications from their diseases, and many are dying despite the best medicines on the market and exposure to world-class health care. So how do we stop this generation from getting sick and dying young?

The news media and health journals have confirmed that the incidence of lifestyle diseases is rapidly rising in the United States of America and other parts of the world. According to the World Health Organization (WHO), millions of deaths occur each year as a result of cardiovascular disease, diabetes, hypertension, cancer, and obesity. In 2012, in the United States, health care spending was $3.8 trillion. Yet people remain sick and die just the same. Cardiovascular disease is the leading cause of death in the United States; in 2011, there were 787,000 deaths as a result of heart disease and stroke. Cancer is the second leading cause of death in America; it is estimated that in 2015, 1,658,320 people were diagnosed with cancer and there were about 589,000 deaths. The incidence of diabetes is at an all-time high. One in every three persons in the United States is either diabetic or prediabetic (meaning the person has higher-than-normal blood sugar levels but not high enough for a diabetes diagnosis). A few years ago ABC News reported that in the year 2020, that number will increase to one in every two persons (50 percent of all Americans will be either diabetic or prediabetic). The incidence of obesity is at an astounding high, with more than two-thirds of American adults being overweight or obese. In children, the number is one in five. If this trend continues, our children's life spans will be much shorter than those of their parents.

The United States is a leader in scientific research, technology, the pharmaceutical industry, large hospitals, and the finest doctors, yet it ranks below many developed countries in health and longevity. Why, then, is America not leading in health and longevity? Could poor lifestyle habits be the leading cause for the health care problem in the United States? Is there any hope for this health care crisis?

The astounding reality of the state of health in my local community has propelled me to become an activist for health and wellness and not merely a good physician. I have become intentional about educating, inspiring, and empowering patients and the community at large to take control of their health destinies.

For the past several years, I have integrated lifestyle medicine into my internal medicine practice, and I have found that these have been my most successful and rewarding years. Patients who carefully follow the principles that I have laid out in my wellness program, the same principles shared with you in my book, *Fourteen Days to Amazing Health*, are now enjoying better health. Many are on a reduced number of medications, and some patients are even off medications altogether. Some patients who were once diabetic now have normal blood sugar without medication as they practice healthy nutrition and regular physical exercise. Other patients are losing weight and feeling great. These actual miracles have propelled me to reach a broader community, and therefore, in 2015, I launched the *Get Healthy with Dr. Cooper* TV show. My message is also in printed form, the *Get Healthy* magazine. There is much joy in knowing that I am touching lives and positively changing the health destinies of tens of thousands of people. It is very rewarding to hear stories like the following: "Hey, Dr. Cooper, I have lost thirty pounds, and I am now ready to proceed with my surgery." Several months ago, a pharmaceutical representative walked into my medical office and said to me, "Dr. Cooper, I lost fifty pounds and am feeling great."

I replied, "What happened? How did you lose the weight?"

He said, "I picked up one of your magazines a few months ago and decided to follow your recommendations and recipes. That was the kickoff." He added that his entire family had changed their lifestyles. Even his three-year-old daughter now frequently asks for kale smoothies.

I have written this book because I want you to have the same opportunity and results that I have seen in those who have followed my wellness program. I want your stories or miracles to be similar or more impacting than those I have shared with you. I want to empower you to change your health destiny. There is absolutely no reason to remain fat, sick, and unhappy for the rest of your life; there is indeed hope beyond the many medications that you take daily. If you are not yet on medications, this book is also for you. The secrets to happiness and long life can be found on these pages.

Fourteen Days to Amazing Health is the answer that you seek as you embark on this journey to a longer, happier, healthier, and more abundant life. Access to this book is like having a personal physician, health coach, and a motivational speaker at your side twenty-four hours a day. Welcome to the journey!

ACKNOWLEDGMENTS

*I*t is impossible to express my sincere thanks to all those who have contributed to this project. However, I will begin by acknowledging my wonderful family. Thank you to my husband of twenty-seven years, Nelson Dockery, who was my biggest support. Nelson, I thank you for your patience and your understanding and for encouraging me to keep focused in order to produce the best book possible. Thank you also to my children, Donnel, Nelson (N. J.), and Dondre; you all have inspired me. Thanks for the vote of confidence and the encouragement to pursue this dream. Donnel, I remember you encouraging me just to do a booklet, and you, N. J., remarking that a cookbook would be much easier to start with. Dondre, you never complained or refused to assist with my never-ending needs to have computer guidance. Thank you all!

I must also thank my mother, Cynthia Ferguson; my sisters, Rosemarie Redway and Carolyn Hannah; and my niece Nickesha for giving your opinions on the initial manuscript and for assisting me with the title of the book.

My heartfelt thanks and deepest appreciation is extended to the staff at Cooper Wellness Center and Cooper Internal Medicine, who have worked tirelessly with this project. Thank you to Maribel Cortina for her work in assisting with the recipes, to Elda Llazos for assisting with the fitness section, and to Donavan Taylor for assisting me with the statistical analysis of the patients' information.

Special thanks to my nephew Christopher Hannah for the role he played in the development of the fitness section of this book. I would also like to thank two very important licensed physical therapists, Vicki Innis and Floyd Courtney, for the time they spent in reviewing and giving valuable advice on the various exercise routines outlined in this book.

To Pastor Randrick Chance, who took time from his busy schedule to share valuable information on how to begin this book project, thank you, and may God continue to bless you and all those lives that you touch. To you Kimasha Williams, my initial editor, words cannot express my sincerest thanks and gratitude for all the hard work that you have put into this project. May God continue to bless you always.

Thanks to those who have assisted me with typing or formatting the manuscript. Jackie and Susana, you both are angels sent to me at the right time. What a blessing you have been!

INTRODUCTION

The Book—What's in It for You?

*G*eorge Garza, a twenty-five-year-old man, walked into my office seeking help. His weight was over 390 pounds, his blood sugar was over 350 (normal blood sugar is between 70 and 105), his hemoglobin A1c was more than 14.0 (normal is between 4.0 and 6.5), and his blood pressure and cholesterol were also above normal. This patient had all the classic features of someone destined for heart disease, renal failure, and early death. His mother, a health care provider, sat in the room with us. She was in disbelief and desperation as she sought help for her son.

As we continued the visit, the patient and his mother revealed to me the underlying causes that led to obesity, diabetes, hypertension, and hyperlipidemia in this young man. At the end of the consultation, I outlined a plan of action, which included the principles outlined in this book, *Fourteen Days to Amazing Health*. In addition to traditional medical therapy, I asked the patient to start on a course of healthy nutrition, which was mostly plan based. He was put on an exercise program, which included daily moderate exercise of at least forty-five minutes to an hour six days a week. He was asked to observe other lifestyle principles, such as managing stress, avoiding tobacco, abstaining from alcohol, and seeking spiritual renewal. At the end of the visit, George and his mother left, motivated to engage in this plan. To date, more than a year later,

George has lost over ninety pounds, his blood sugar is now normal, his last hemoglobin A1c was 5.3, and his blood pressure and cholesterol have also improved. Even though George has had setbacks, he continues to maintain a healthy diet, the weight has stayed off, his blood sugar remains controlled, and he is motivated to continue forward on this journey to a happier, healthier, and longer life.

Your story might be different from George's; however, I hope that you are inspired to explore the information in this book. *Fourteen Days to Amazing Health* is a jump-start program. It takes a unique approach in addressing the whole person. My program is laid out in a simple fashion, step by step, day by day, which will give you easy coaching as you follow along. The program is an evidence-based plan, one that I have used for many years to help patients improve or reverse chronic illnesses. As you continue to read, you will notice that I have shared some of those patients' stories throughout the book.

Though my program does require your commitment, you will agree with me that the solution to our health care crisis is not another pill. The health care industry and researchers now realize that in most cases, chronic diseases develop as a result of engaging in unhealthy lifestyle habits, and thus these diseases can be significantly improved, prevented, or reversed with healthy lifestyle choices. Researchers are now confirming that reducing the intake of animal products and refined foods and increasing the intake of fresh fruits, vegetables, and whole grains, coupled with daily physical exercise, could greatly improve, prevent, or reverse some of these chronic lifestyle diseases, such as diabetes, coronary artery disease, obesity, hypertension, and even some cancers.

An article was published in the *Journal of the American Medical Association* in July 2013 showing that the leading risk factor of early death in the United States and other Western countries was the dietary factor (poor diet). Let us reflect on this fact. The number-one risk factor for chronic disease and early death is food. The type of food that you consume either promotes good health or increases the risk of chronic diseases. I am thoroughly in agreement with Hippocrates, one of the founders of medicine, who rightly states, "Let food be thy medicine and medicine be thy food."

For the last several years I have been using "food as medicine" with my patients, and they are indeed enjoying much better health. Many of these patients have lost weight and reduced medications. Some have even become free of previously diagnosed diseases and prescribed medications. They are happier, healthier, and more fulfilled. As I witnessed the many health miracles in the lives of my patients, resulting from a healthy lifestyle, my desire to touch more lives has grown stronger each day. Patients once categorized as obese are now in the healthy weight category, and those once prescribed medications—for life—have put their disease in retreat.

I also want you to have the opportunity to improve your health! I suggest you take the test at the back of this book and assess your lifestyle. Is your lifestyle healthy? Are you taking too many medications? What is your health goal for the future? You do have an alternative that you probably are not aware of. It is my desire that as you read and adopt the principles laid out in this book that your health story will be similar to those of the patients you will learn about in this book.

As you travel along this journey with me, you will be given health facts on the optimal nutrition and I will share with you the most recent research information on the health benefits of the foods that you will be enjoying. You will be asked to make adjustment in your eating habits and to incorporate new food items into your diet. A suggested daily meal plan is laid out in the book with healthy and tasty recipes. Now please note that I will not be placing you on a diet. This is a way of life. You will be educated on the reasons why these foods are necessary in your diet so that you can make this a lifestyle that you can live with.

There is a wealth of research now confirming that regular physical exercise is as important as embracing healthy nutrition. With this in mind, I have laid out in this book a full fitness program, which is appropriate for all fitness levels. In other words, my book, *Fourteen Days to Amazing Health*, will provide you with the information you need in order to engage in meaningful regular physical exercise.

In order to obtain whole-person health and wellness, it is of vital importance that we address other healthy lifestyle factors, such as the mind-body connection, optimism, negative emotions, social connectedness, adequate rest, and spiritual renewal. I have addressed all of these in my book. Many people are unaware of some simple natural remedies that are essential for good health. Let us look at water, for example. I was giving a lecture recently to a group of people, and I spoke about the health benefits of water. I emphasized that water is important to treat kidney stones, constipation, dehydration, headache, and fatigue and even to prevent venous blood clots. The audience was amazed. Many times, as health care providers, we take the simple things for granted; however, if we empower people like you, then we will be doing more justice to our health care system by preventing chronic diseases and thus promoting healthy people, healthy communities, and a healthy nation.

I urge you today to define your health goals and then make the decision to commit to this program. I know for a fact that it will change the course of your health and life forever. Many have walked this path before. They have written beautiful and amazing health stories. You too have a story to write, so come along with me as I hold your hand and assist you in writing your story of health miracles. Practicing medicine now has become more gratifying to me as I witness lives being changed as people become educated, inspired, and empowered to make healthy lifestyle modifications.

PART 1

Amazing Health Facts

CHAPTER 1

Change Belief and Live

_T_here is a general belief that diseases like diabetes, hypertension, coronary artery disease, and cerebrovascular disease result only from genetic predispositions—meaning that if your parents or family members suffer from one or more of these chronic diseases, you are at risk for developing the same illnesses. While this notion is partially true, scientists are also well aware that these diseases can be delayed, inhibited, accelerated, or altogether prevented, depending on your lifestyle.

Several years ago, I had a very interesting encounter with a young couple. The wife was insistent that her obese husband change his eating habits and start a regular exercise program. The husband adamantly refused, stating that all of his family members were obese as well as diabetic. He was, therefore, convinced that this would also be his destiny. Thus, he saw no value in changing his lifestyle. It is a mistake to think that health is predestined. Health is a choice! And what we know for certain is that poor health accelerates the aging process and can eventually lead to early death.

People are consuming inappropriately large amounts of calories that they are unable to use. The extra calories, if not expended or burned during physical activity, get stored as glycogen, which is later converted into adipose or what we know as fat tissue. This, of course, leads to obesity. Several key environmental and cultural factors have come together over the course of the past few decades to markedly increase the risk of both active and passive overeating. Chief among these are the increased availability and promotion of cheap, energy-dense diets, usually high in fat, and the transition toward extremely sedentary lifestyles. Thus, overeating, poor food choices, and lack of physical activity will definitely lead to obesity. Obesity increases your risk of diabetes, hypertension, obstructive sleep apnea syndrome, and arthritis. If you are suffering from any or a combination of these diseases, you are aging faster than you should.

But for now, let's focus on diabetes.

It is a known fact that obese patients are at increased risk for insulin resistance. These obese patients are unable to effectively metabolize glucose. Consequently, they become predisposed to developing type 2 diabetes. Having diabetes then places these patients at a greater risk for a host of other diseases, such as coronary artery disease, stroke, renal failure, and blindness; it is believed that 70 percent of all children and 35 percent of adults in the United States are obese. By 2030, 42 percent of adults will be obese. A few years ago, a nationwide survey conducted by the National Institutes of Health cited the city in which I currently reside, McAllen-Mission, Texas, as the fattest in the United States, with just under 40 percent of our population obese. I was astounded after reading this information. As a health care provider, I am acutely aware that it is no longer acceptable to only treat these chronic illnesses; it is most important to prevent, retard, or stop their development by educating the community with the intent to effectuate change in behavior and lifestyle. As a practicing physician for over twenty-five years, I have become uncomfortable with only prescribing an antihypertensive pill for a twenty-two-year-old young man with a blood pressure of 160/90, a weight of 300 pounds, and a BMI of 50. I know that I will serve him better if I am able to give him a plan to achieve lifestyle changes and a way to lose weight. This will result in improved health, and he will have a better chance to lead a normal life.

So here is the first step to changing your health destiny. First, believe that there is hope beyond diabetes, hypertension, obesity, and heart disease. You hold the key to your health success, and you do not have to live with this disease or live in fear of developing it later in life. If you already have any of these diseases and find yourself taking many medications, you can still have hope. I have seen so many patients who were once dependent on multiple drugs see a decrease or complete elimination of their medication after a change in lifestyle. You too can experience this freedom to good health. But you first have to believe that it is possible.

CHAPTER 2

The Health Program You Need

*O*ver the past several years, I have seen patients frustrated with their health and their health care providers. These patients are usually on many drugs but still have poor health with the constant lingering question in mind, *Am I destined to live this way for the rest of my life?* Are you one of those individuals with this fear? Are you thinking that there may not be any hope for your particular disease? Often, patients are told that once they become diabetic, they will be on medication for the rest of their lives. Have you heard that before? Well, let me help you eliminate that myth from your mind. There are many diseases that are strongly influenced by the way we live our lives or by the choices we make. Choosing not to smoke, to embrace a healthy diet, to be physically active, and to live without anger and hate can significantly impact your health.

I am sure that you have heard this *excuse* before: "Well, diabetes runs in my family, so I know that I will get diabetes eventually." Do you identify with that statement? Don't feel bad; most people think the same way. During my many years of practicing medicine, I have spent a considerable amount of time educating people on the root causes of chronic diseases, such as diabetes, hypertension, obesity, heart disease, arthritis, sleep apnea, and some cancers, just to name a few. Poor lifestyle habits will shape your health destiny, not your family history or your genes. *The way we live our lives and the choices that we make can significantly influence our health. Someone rightly said that our genes load the gun, but our lifestyle pulls the trigger.*

In the United States, type 2 diabetes has become a public health crisis. Do you know that 80 to 90 percent of people with this disease could successfully cure themselves and get off medication just by simply changing their lifestyle? I know you are probably in disbelief. I have success stories from many of my patients who have met with this success. If you are a person with type 2 diabetes or other chronic diseases, then upon completion of this book, you will have the secrets to a new and healthier lifestyle. You too will have a success story to share.

Meet the Gonzalezes, mother and son. Mrs. Gonzalez came to me at age seventy-seven with diabetes, hypertension, arthritis, depression, and obesity. She was very frustrated with the number of pills she was taking yet still being in poor health. The constant knee pain made it very difficult to get around so she had to use a walker for support. I remember a particular visit with Mrs. Gonzalez; she was frustrated with her health status. I felt her anger and hopelessness. She was in search of something more than just another pill or a quick and easy fix.

It is not unfair to say that most of my colleagues, as doctors, find it easier to medicate or just manage the disease. Recently, the focus in health care is slowly changing to prevention of diseases, but only very few health care providers actually address the root causes of these chronic diseases. Well, during this particular visit with Mrs. Gonzalez, I offered her a new approach to treating her overall medical issues, which has dramatically changed her life.

I asked Mrs. Gonzalez to come in for weekly educational seminars where the focus was on healthy nutrition and regular physical exercise, as well as other important healthy lifestyle principles. She slowly began to change her diet and became more physically active. However, there were times when she became discouraged. Adopting this new lifestyle was indeed difficult for her. But she wanted a new and healthier body. This was her goal, so she continued to focus on the reward. A few weeks into the program, the challenge became too great. The change that she was hoping to experience just was not happening, so she began to avoid me. She would attend the weekly lectures but quickly exit the office without visiting with me. Mrs. Gonzales later revealed to me that the breakthrough happened when she truly began to adhere to the healthy diet plan.

After successfully completing twelve weeks in the wellness program, Mrs. Gonzalez lost thirty-five pounds, she was now off the diabetes medication and decreased the number of medications for hypertension and pain. Most important, she was feeling younger, healthier, and happier; she had less knee pain and was not dependent on her walking cane anymore. One year later, she has lost about fifty-six pounds and her blood sugar remains normal off medication.

And what about her son? He was not my patient; however, he took his mother to the weekly seminars, listened to the advice, and began to change his lifestyle. Obviously, he also has a success story. He lost twenty-five pounds, and because of his improved health, his doctor reduced his high blood pressure medications.

I enjoy sharing Mrs. Gonzalez's story when I do seminars. I think many people can be encouraged by this seventy-seven-year-old woman who decided that she no longer wanted to be sick with diabetes, depression, and obesity or use a walking cane. I truly believe if you have the burning desire, drive, and focus to change, similar to Mrs. Gonzalez, then success is just around the corner. I must tell you that I have many similar stories of patients who have lost weight and are enjoying better health off medications for diabetes, hypertension, high cholesterol, and even for heart disease. I will continue to introduce them to you in this book.

You may now be wondering. *What is the secret to these patients' success?*

Thousands of years ago, Hippocrates discovered what many researchers are only now concluding—that food is the number-one risk factor for many diseases. How much more serious is the Hippocrates quote today, "Let food be thy medicine and medicine be thy food." In recent years, health researchers have identified health-risk foods, such as refined grains, sugar, salt, red and processed meats, and dairy. Additionally, a low intake of fruits, vegetables, legumes, seeds, and nuts also poses risks to our health. With these observations, researchers are confirming Hippocrates's notion that the consumption of certain foods will promote good health.

Now for the big question: *Why has my health care provider not shared this with me?*

The health care industry is now realizing that in order to create a healthy nation, we need healthy individuals who are educated on preventing and protecting themselves from chronic diseases now known as lifestyle diseases. The key to this success is not just to manage the symptoms of these diseases; the true secret is to get to the root causes. Poor food choices, inactivity, stress, lack of sleep, and lack of family connectedness, as well as lack of hope, are some of the major root causes of the current health crisis facing us today.

Now the health care industry is taking a new look at how to address this crisis. And here is the secret behind my patients' success story. The patients with chronic diseases, such as diabetes, hypertension, obesity, heart disease, and high cholesterol, enroll in a twelve-week program and are given a diet of fruits, vegetables, nuts, seeds, and whole grains. They are encouraged to exercise for at least thirty minutes a day for six days per week. The program encourages two main meals a day with breakfast being the largest meal, a moderate-sized lunch, and a light, small snack for supper; this last snack is taken at or about five in the evening. The participants in this program are asked to increase their water intake and to reduce the intake of soda and concentrated fruit juices, sugary drinks, and coffee. The program also focuses on stress management; the patients are encouraged to read the Bible to obtain an understanding of the Creator's plan for their optimal health.

I am currently practicing internal medicine, and not all of my patients are willing to enter this program for a lifestyle change. However, the patients with the best results, those who are actually getting off medications, those with better blood sugar and blood pressure control, and those who are less short of breath while exercising, are the patients who have integrated lifestyle medicine with their medical care. As a physician who has been practicing medicine since 1991, I can honestly tell you that I am indeed much more satisfied with my profession now than ever before. I want my patients to get well, stay well, and enjoy their God-given potential. I want you, the readers of this book, to obtain the same benefits that so many of my patients have enjoyed and are currently enjoying.

The program is very simple. Start by listing all the fruits, vegetables, whole grains, nuts, and seeds that you enjoy eating. Then learn how to consume these foods in a healthier manner, using less fat, sugar, and salt. While learning how to prepare healthy meals for yourself and your family, you may consider healthy restaurant choices, such as bean burritos, pizza using only vegetable toppings without the cheese, pasta with marinara sauce, or a tofu dish at an Asian restaurant. Salads are also great choices; just leave out the meats and remember to use low-fat dressings. If you add beans, peas, or whole grains like quinoa and nuts, then you have a great dish. How could I forget vegetable soup? This is my favorite! Soup is a great way to fill up without packing on the calories. For breakfast, I suggest cooked oats, whole-grain cereals with nondairy milk, fruits, granola, or whole-grain bread with nut butter or leftover beans made into a spread. Now, would you agree that changing to a healthier lifestyle is not all that difficult?

CHAPTER 3

Establishing Good Habits and Meal Planning

*I*t is important to remove bad habits from your daily routine. Nonetheless, you will agree with me that changing habits is very difficult. Imagine enjoying a particular dish for breakfast every day for forty years. It is not just your favorite breakfast meal but also your great-grandmother's recipe! After learning that this tasteful traditional breakfast could endanger your health, you decide to eliminate it from your breakfast regime. Now let's be honest, this change will be difficult.

So what do you do when faced with a difficult decision to change to a healthier lifestyle as you seek a more abundant life? For some people, this may be a desperate choice to hang on to life. I want you to understand that an early choice to live healthy will delay illnesses.

As I work with people who attend my seminars, I find that some will adopt the change easily while others will experience a real struggle. I must share with you the story of Mr. Cantu, a fifty-eight-year-old Hispanic man who has been my patient for many years. I met Mr. Cantu with diabetes, hypertension, obesity, high cholesterol, severe knee pain, and a walking cane for support.

Mr. Cantu entered my lifestyle program because he wanted to improve his health, but he just could not put the old habits aside. He continued to eat processed foods and a high-fat diet, he was not engaging in physical exercise as instructed; his blood sugar remained high, and his weight was not changing. This continued for a while. Then one day, he walked into my office as a new person; his weight was trending down, and his blood sugar was normal. He was indeed a different man. I was eager to hear his story, and with much enthusiasm, I asked, "Mr. Cantu, what did you do differently?"

He said, "Dr. Cooper, I have been praying and reading my Bible more, and this has given me the strength to make the changes that I need to make."

Meditation, prayer, and seeking divine intervention may be what you need to do in order to be empowered to make a healthy lifestyle change that will last for a lifetime. I am confident that you can change your thinking and behavior and take an active part in improving your entire life. Change is usually difficult but not impossible. You must first be mentally ready to make the change. You will need to assess your health risks, determine your goals, and then map out the desired path that you will pursue to achieve these goals. This is the first step toward true and lasting health.

According to the experts, your brain is wired by your habitual actions. When you repeatedly do a task—especially for many years—your brain maps pathways that cause you to perform that act without even thinking. However, the good news is you can rewire your brain simply by replacing actions that lead to poor overall health with positive ones. So you don't have to be stuck in neutral.

Again, to break a bad habit, you need to replace the bad habit with a good one. I understand that this is more difficult than it sounds, more so if you have been practicing this bad habit for many years. It is even more complicated if you have sustained an injury or had a major, life-changing event that got you off track in your life. There is indeed a very intimate and powerful connection between the mind and the body. Research has shown that every thought we process, whether positive or negative, has a physiological response in our bodies. Negative emotions, such as the feeling of anger, hate, or lack of forgiveness, will increase the risk of diseases like hypertension, heart disease, stroke, and even death. Positive thoughts, such as happiness and hope, in contrast are essential for the development of healthy behaviors and thus a happier and longer life.

Take heart. You can make it! As long as you have life, there is hope! Here is a formula for you to try. For a minimum of three times a day, for seven consecutive days, stop one bad habit and replace it with the right habit. You will see enormous changes. You can actually bring about change in your brain by introducing a good habit perpetually for as few as seven days.

The first place to begin your change process is in your eating habits. As you continue to read this book, you will be introduced to my sample meal plan. The best part is a fourteen-day meal plan that is provided for you to follow. This will assist you in reinforcing changes in your eating habits. You will need purpose in your heart to stick with the plan! You must remove things from your sight that may tempt you to relapse. To ensure success, stock up with healthy foods that you enjoy. When you have gone through this fourteen-day period, you will be equipped to take more control and design your own meal plans. As you contemplate building good habits that will promote a healthier you, here are some foods to avoid:

- all processed grains (white rice, white bread, white pasta, quick oats)
- red and processed meats (beef, pork, hot dog, ham, bacon, salami, sausage, deli meats)
- snack foods (chips, fries, candy bars)
- soda or sugary drinks
- dairy and eggs
- animal fat and oil
- coffee and caffeinated drinks

- alcohol
- extra salt

You should consume more of the following:

- whole grains (brown rice, whole wheat bread and pasta, barley, rolled oats, quinoa, rye)
- fruits and vegetables
- legumes and tubers (peas, beans, lentil, chickpeas, sweet potato)
- nuts and seeds
- water

CHAPTER 4

Healthy Food Pantry

*Y*our kitchen pantry should have the very best foods to ensure the proper health for you and your family. The best way to be healthy is to stock up on the healthy foods that you enjoy. The following are recommended food lists by category. Feel free to add those healthy foods that you enjoy. You can purchase everything listed below at your local grocer. Natural, raw, and organic is ideal.

Grains
barley
brown rice
bulgur wheat
couscous
millet
multigrain cereal
oats (old-fashioned, rolled)
rye
spelt
quinoa
tortillas
whole-grain bread
whole-grain flours
whole-grain pastas
wild rice

Flours
cornmeal
whole wheat
wheat bran
oat
chickpea
brown rice
rye
barley
spelt
soy
vital gluten wheat germ

Legumes
black beans
black-eyed peas
garbanzo beans (chickpeas)
navy beans
kidney beans
pinto beans
lima beans
lentils
red beans
soybeans
split peas
peanuts

Nuts and Seeds
almond
cashew
chia seeds

coconut

pecans

pumpkin seeds

sesame seeds

sunflower seeds

walnuts

flaxseeds

whole flaxseed

Nut Butters

almond butter

cashew butter

peanut butter

tahini

Dried Fruits

cranberry

dates

figs

prunes

raisins

Dried Herbs & Spices

allspice

sage

basil

rosemary

cayenne pepper

Italian seasoning

celery seeds

cumin

curry powder

onion powder

garlic powder

ground cinnamon

McKay's chicken-style seasoning

Mrs. Dash herbal seasoning

nutritional yeast flakes

turmeric

oregano

coriander

sea salt

cinnamon

Fruits and Vegetables

fresh fruits and vegetables of all varieties and colors

Canned Items

beans

light coconut milk

olives

tomato paste (sauce)

pimentos

vegetable broth

Equipment

blender

food processor

waffle iron

CHAPTER 5

Fill Up with Whole Grains

$\mathcal{H}$ave you noticed lately that the world is demanding more information on whole grains like quinoa, barley, brown rice, and oats? There is also a surge in the consumption of these grains. What do these grains have in common? Did you know that consuming a few servings of whole grain weekly may reduce your risk for coronary artery disease and may help to prevent, improve, or reverse diabetes? What is so special about these grains? Are they medicinal? Should you fill up your pantry with them?

GRAINS DEFINED

Grains are an essential component of a healthy diet. Most people consume grains daily. Grains produce a significant part of the energy source in their diets. Grains also provide fiber, iron, minerals, and various types of nutrients that are important for proper body function.

The issue with grains is the type or the quality. Are the grains you consume whole grains (unprocessed), or are they refined (processed)? This is an important question to ask yourself when you think of purchasing grains.

Now let's look at the difference between whole grains and refined grains. A grain is composed of three main parts:

- bran, which is the fibrous shell and contains the most nutrients
- endosperm, also known as the kernel, makes up the bulk of the grain and contains a small amount of vitamins and minerals
- germ, which is the smallest part of the grain but contains lots of nutrients and healthy fats.

These three vital components make up the whole grain. Usually when the grain is processed, the bran and the germ are removed, leaving behind the endosperm, which is mainly carbohydrates with few vital nutrients.

THE ANATOMY OF THE GRAIN

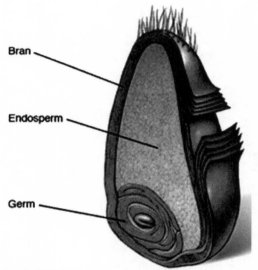

Some examples of whole grain products are brown rice, wheat berries, quinoa, barley, rye, bulgur, millet, and corn.

WHAT MAKES THESE GRAINS SPECIAL?

1. Whole grains contain a higher content of essential nutrients, such as vitamin E, thiamine, iron, and magnesium, as well as fiber and antioxidants.

2. Refined grains are finer in texture and have a longer shelf life; however, the milling process has removed iron, B complex vitamins, and fiber.

3. With enriched grains, certain nutrients that were removed were added back to the grain. Enriched grains are still inferior to whole grains in terms of the quality of nutrients they provide as well as the health benefits that these grains offer (see USDA Chosemyplate.gov/grains). Some grains are fortified, which means nutrients that don't occur naturally in the food were added in.

Dietary guidelines for Americans recommend that at least half of all the grains you eat are whole grains. It is therefore important to read the labels carefully to ensure that you are obtaining food with the highest amount of nutrients required to promote optimal health.

HEALTH BENEFITS OF CONSUMING THE ENTIRE GRAIN (WHOLE GRAIN)

The higher fiber content in whole grains assists in slowing glucose absorption. This will decrease the glucose spike seen in diabetics and therefore will lead to better glucose control. It may even lead to a reversal of diabetes. Fiber has more bulk. It remains longer in the stomach. This keeps you feeling fuller longer, which then decreases the need to snack between meals. Consuming foods high in fiber, such as whole grains, is a great way to lose weight and maintain a healthier weight. Fiber is also great to lower LDL cholesterol. It gives bulk to the stool, which is important for regular bowel movements. Regular bowel movements reduce the risk of constipation and the formation of diverticulosis, which results from high pressure within the large intestines producing bulging pouches in the lining of the bowel.

Whole grains are nutrient dense and calorie poor in comparison to processed grains. This means that there are more protein, vitamins, minerals, and phytonutrients in whole grains than in processed grains; therefore, the consumption of whole grains provides greater health benefits. Processed grains, in contrast, are depleted of some fiber, vitamins, minerals, and phytonutrients. These grains are left with mostly the carbohydrate portion. Consuming a diet of mostly processed grains may increase your risk for obesity, diabetes, and heart disease.

Whole Grains and Heart Disease

Did you know that eating whole grains instead or refined grains could substantially lower total cholesterol, low-density lipoprotein (LDL or bad) cholesterol, triglycerides, and insulin levels and may even lower your risk of forming blood clots? A growing body of evidence now shows a link between better heart health and the consumption of whole grains.

In the Harvard-based *Nurses' Health Study*, results showed women who ate two to three servings of whole-grain products each day were 30 percent less likely to have a heart attack or die from heart disease over a ten-year period than those who ate less than one serving per day. In another study, a meta-analysis of seven major studies, cardiovascular disease (heart attack, stroke, or the need for a procedure to bypass or open a clogged artery) was 21 percent less likely in people who ate two and a half servings or more of whole-grain products per day compared to those who ate less than two servings a week.

Whole Grains and Type 2 Diabetes

Over the past several years, we have seen a surge in the obesity and diabetes crises, which parallel the intake of processed foods and fats.

However, more recent findings from various research studies suggest that switching from white rice to brown rice, for example, could help lower diabetes risk. Results from the *Nurses' Health Study* showed individuals who ate five or more servings of white rice per week had a 17 percent greater risk of diabetes than those who ate white rice less than five times per month. Those who ate the most brown rice (two or more servings per week) had an 11 percent lower risk of diabetes than those who rarely ate brown rice (less than one time per month).

If you are a diabetic, then whole grains should be your friend at mealtime. You have probably heard the terms *good carbs* and *bad carbs*. Well, whole grains are the *good carbs*. The consumption of whole grains not only allows for a slower absorption of glucose to the blood, thus blunting blood sugar spikes, but these grains contain fewer calories so you can eat more with less risk of weight gain. Additionally, whole grains remain longer in the stomach; therefore, you will feel full longer, which usually eliminates the desire to snack.

All these positive factors will promote weight loss or the maintenance of a healthy weight. If you have type 2 diabetes, then losing the extra weight could propel you on your way to reversing diabetes or significantly decreasing the amount of medications that you are currently taking. If you are prediabetic, having a healthy weight will decrease your risk of poor insulin function and subsequently type 2 diabetes.

Permit me to introduce you to another patient of mine. George, at seventy-two years old, was morbidly obese with diabetes and high blood pressure. He came to me with various medications to control these diseases; however, after less than three months on a diet high in whole grains, vegetables, and legumes, coupled with daily exercise, George was able to lose more than thirty pounds. He is now off all medications. His blood sugar remains normal. He is very happy, and he continues to share his new lifestyle secrets with friends and family. George is the cook at home; he revealed to me recently that he has the other family members eating the way he does.

Fiber Content in Whole Grains

Types of Whole Grains (1 Cup Cooked)	Grams of Fiber
rye	25
sorghum	12
spelt	8
bulgur	8
farro	7
barley	6
whole wheat pasta	6
amaranth	5
buckwheat	5
corn kernel	5
quinoa	5
brown rice	4
oats	4
wheat	4
wild rice	3
millet	2
whole wheat bread	2
white bread	1

Usual fiber recommendations are thirty to thirty-eight grams a day for men, twenty-five grams a day for women between eighteen and fifty years of age, and twenty-one grams a day for women fifty-one and older.

WHAT ABOUT CANCER?

The data on whole grain consumption and cancer is not very clear; however, I am sure that you have heard before that a diet high in fiber and low in red meats could provide protection from colon cancer. The consumption of whole grains will help maximize the fiber content in the diet, which could lower your risk of colon cancer. Whole grains ferment in the colon through the action of bacteria in the colon. This action produces colon-cancer-preventing short-chain fatty acids.

Results from a five-year study of five hundred thousand men and women showed eating whole grains, separate from dietary fiber, was moderately associated with lower colorectal cancer risk. Now tell me, who wants to be at risk for any cancer? So why take the risk, when whole grains are so readily available and easy to incorporate into the diet?

HYPERTENSION AND WHOLE GRAINS

Researchers now believe that a healthy lifestyle and dietary measures may prevent many chronic diseases, such as hypertension. In the *Women's Health Study*, researchers concluded that women who consumed at least four servings of whole grains daily had a 23 percent reduced risk of developing hypertension compared to those who consumed less than one-half of that daily.

Other studies have supported the use of whole grains in controlling hypertension. The *2010 Dietary Guideline for Americans* suggests the dietary approach to stopping hypertension (DASH diet) of which whole grain is an integral part.

Ways to Increase Your Consumption of Whole Grains

1. A "whole grain" stamp on food items does not always mean healthy grain; therefore, learn to read food labels carefully and purchase those items that are 100 percent whole grain.
2. Where possible, use whole grain rather than whole grain products, for example, choose wheat berries over whole wheat crackers.
3. Have oatmeal at breakfast.
4. Enjoy popcorn without the butter as a snack.
5. Serve corn on the cob as a side dish.
6. Serve brown or wild rice at mealtime.
7. Choose whole-grain bread, rolls, buns, and so on.
8. Use whole wheat pasta
9. Use other whole grains, such as barley, rye, and quinoa.
10. Add barley or brown rice to your soups.

I am well aware that making healthy lifestyle changes may sometimes appear daunting; however, you can begin by taking simple steps, such as those just mentioned, as you continue your journey to good health and longevity.

CHAPTER 6

Fats—the Good and the Bad

$\mathcal{C}$ontrary to the belief that a diet devoid of fat is the best, fat is actually an essential component of a healthy and balanced diet. Dietary fat is a major energy source, and fat supports cell growth. In addition, fat helps protect our organs and aids in keeping our body warm. Other important functions of dietary fat include aiding in absorption of certain nutrients, such as fat-soluble vitamins (A, D, E, K), and producing important hormones. Fat is also needed to build cell membranes, the vital exterior of each cell, and the sheaths surrounding the nerves. It is essential for blood clotting and muscle movement. Without an appropriate amount of fat in the diet, the body will not function efficiently. It is therefore fair to say that the main problems with dietary fats is the type and amount that you consume. The type of fat is directly related to its source.

Now Let's Focus on Types of Fats

You have probably heard the phrase "not all fats are created equal." Some fats are healthier than others. Healthy fats, also known as "good fats," are usually obtained from plant sources. On the other hand, unhealthy fats, or "bad fats," are usually derived from animal-based products or manufactured by humans (trans fat). When healthy vegetable oil is hydrogenated to become semisolid fat, this is called *trans fatty acid*. This type of fat is very unhealthy.

UNHEALTHY OR BAD FATS

Saturated fat is usually derived from animal products, such as meat, milk, cheese, and eggs. Coconut and palm oils are plant sources of saturated fats. Trans fat is produced when healthy vegetable oil is hydrogenated to form semisolid or solid fats. These fats are unhealthy or "bad" fats. Saturated fat has been shown to increase total blood cholesterol level and low density-lipoprotein (LDL) or bad cholesterol levels. High LDL levels will increase your risk for heart disease and possibly type 2 diabetes, especially when combined with a diet high in refined carbohydrates. It is therefore safe to say that a diet high in meat or other animal products will influence your cholesterol level. Of course the level of saturated fat is directly related to the fat content of the animal product. I am sure that at this point you might be wondering how much of animal products you could consume and still keep your cholesterol at a normal level. Some studies recommend the consumption of lean meats not more than twice weekly while others suggest total abstinence from all animal products for optimal health.

Like saturated fat, trans fat could also increase LDL (bad cholesterol) levels while suppressing HDL (good cholesterol) levels. Trans fat, therefore, can increase your risk of heart disease three times as much as saturated fat intake. Trans fats create inflammation, which is linked to heart disease, stroke, and other chronic diseases. Trans fats may contribute to insulin resistance, which increases the risk of type 2 diabetes. Researchers from the Harvard School of Public Health indicate that trans fats can harm health. Even in small amounts of 2 percent daily, they will increase the risk of heart disease by 23 percent.

HEALTHY OR GOOD FATS

Healthy fats are usually obtained from plant sources, such as nuts, seeds, olives, and avocado. Fats obtained from plants are monounsaturated and polyunsaturated. The famous omega-3 and omega-6 fatty acids are examples of polyunsaturated fats. These fats will lower the LDL (bad) cholesterol level and will increase the HDL (good) cholesterol level. Plant fats are usually liquid at room temperature; however, as mentioned earlier, when these oils are hydrogenated, they become semisolid at room temperature. This process produces trans fat, which is very harmful to health. Examples of trans fat are found in butter and shortening and in cookies, cakes, and other baked goods.

It is quite alarming to know that only a small percentage of people in our society consume nuts and seeds on a regular basis. Nuts and seeds make up a very important part of a healthy diet. These foods provide not only essential nutrients, such as protein and fiber, but also the good healthy fats that the body needs for disease prevention and maintaining good health. Nuts and seeds are natural hunger-busters, not only because of their fat content but also because of their protein and fiber content. All nuts contain fiber, which helps lower cholesterol while anchoring a person's blood sugar.

Consuming a handful of nuts and seeds five times a week has significant health benefits. This provides a great source of dietary fiber. One ounce of flaxseeds will provide 7.5 grams of fiber, while an ounce of almond nut will provide 3.5 grams of fiber. As mentioned before, undigested fiber adds bulk to the stool, which promotes regular bowel movements. Fiber also helps to slow the rate of digestion, which consequently decreases the rise in sugar in the blood. This action promotes better glucose control in diabetics and can lead to diabetes reversal.

Most nuts, especially peanuts, contain slimming nutrients. Peanuts can be considered the unsung heroes when it comes to building lean muscle mass, because they contain the nonessential amino acid L-arginine. It is being studied for its ability to decrease body fat while helping to build lean muscle mass at the same time. Nuts also contain a wide array of antioxidants and vital minerals that most people lack, including the following:

- ✓ calcium
- ✓ chromium
- ✓ iron
- ✓ manganese
- ✓ zinc
- ✓ selenium, which is important for many physiological and metabolic functions

If you are trying to lose fat, eating fats for weight loss is so important! It might seem counterintuitive, but not getting enough good quality fats along with other vital nutrients in your diet can sabotage your weight-loss efforts. Nuts and seeds provide the body with cholesterol-free fat. This type of fat will therefore promote heart health as well as good overall health.

Monounsaturated Fats

Studies show that eating foods rich in monounsaturated fats improves blood cholesterol levels, which decreases heart disease risk. These fatty acids have also been associated with better insulin levels and blood sugar control. In the *Nurses' Health Study*, it was reported that women who ate five units of nuts (one unit equivalent to 1 ounce of nuts) a week had a significantly lower risk of total coronary heart disease than women who never ate nuts or who ate less than one unit monthly.

Polyunsaturated fats

Evidence shows that consuming foods high in polyunsaturated fats improves blood cholesterol levels and decreases the risk of heart disease.

Omega-3 Fatty Acids

Omega-3s are one type of polyunsaturated fat that is especially beneficial to the heart. They have been shown to decrease the risk of coronary artery disease. Plant food sources of omega-3 include walnuts, sunflower seeds, flaxseed, and chia seeds.

TIPS TO ENSURE THE INTAKE OF HEALTHY FATS

Do not be fooled; fat is essential for good health. The trick, however, is in the type of fat that you choose to consume. Here are the secrets to eating fat and staying trim and healthy:

- Use vegetable oil instead of butter, margarine, or lard. You must be cautious of the fact that too much oil will lead to excess calories and consequently this may lead to obesity. While eliminating solid fats from the diet, remember to use oil sparingly.
- Use nuts, seeds, olives, and avocado. Strive to consume a handful of nuts and two to three tablespoonfuls of sesame, flax, or pumpkins seeds daily. Nuts and seeds will provide not only good fats but also a high content of protein, fiber, iron, calcium, zinc, copper, vitamin E, and other nutrients.
- Avoid animal products. Meat, dairy, and cheese are the top sources of unhealthy fat. These foods are high in saturated fat and calories but low in nutrients and fiber.
- Avoid partially hydrogenated oils. These are trans fats seen usually in baked or fried foods, so learn to read food labels well.

Research has shown that the type of fat you consume could either increase the risk of diseases or protect you from diseases, such as type 2 diabetes, coronary artery disease, and even cancer. Therefore, here is my suggestion: first, reduce or eliminate your consumption of saturated fats and cholesterol. Foods highest in saturated fats and cholesterol are meats, pizza, butter, whole milk, cakes, eggs, pastries, and dairy products. Second, eliminate all trans fats from your diet. Third, replace these bad fats with nuts, seeds, olives, and canola, soy, and sunflower oils. Nut butters are also acceptable.

However, be reminded that oils are processed food, and like everything else, they must be used in moderation. Even though vegetable oils are loaded with polyunsaturated fats, which are great to lower cholesterol, they are high in calories—one tablespoon of olive oil provides 120 calories. Therefore, consuming lots of oil in your diet in whatever form, whether by deep-frying or on your salad, is not good for your health.

Some of you reading this book might be wondering if it is possible to prepare tasty meals without the use of oil. The answer is yes! There are many simple, delicious, and amazing recipes in this book that you will enjoy. These recipes can be created using very little or no oil. You and your family will enjoy these recipes as you continue on your quest for a longer and happier life.

CHAPTER 7

Legumes—Love Them or Hate Them

*M*ost people are not aware of the importance of peas, beans, lentils, and other legumes in their diet. The legume family is a staple in the traditional diets of many countries around the world. However, it is usually less appreciated in the typical Western diet. Legumes are inexpensive and an excellent source of protein, complex carbohydrates, minerals, vitamins, fiber, and antioxidants and an ideal substitute for meat. Consequently, legumes are usually regarded as the "poor man's meat."

However, while animal proteins are high in saturated fats, legumes are free of them. In most cases, one cup of peas or beans contains about fifteen grams of protein, which is 33 percent of the daily requirement for females and about 28 percent for males. Beans are very high in fiber and low on the glycemic index. They give you about a third of your daily fiber requirements in just a half cup (at around 190 calories) and are also good sources of magnesium (important for heart health) and potassium (crucial for muscle function and hydration). Like berries and greens, beans are in the running for the top antioxidant-rich foods, a little known fact. Kidney and red beans rank highest, with black beans following close behind. Black beans are especially good for digestive tract health and have been studied in the context of colon cancer.

Types of Legumes

There are many different types of legumes; they are divided into immature legumes and mature legumes. Immature legumes are often referred to as fresh legumes. This includes all types of edible pod beans and peas and shell beans that have not yet been dried. Here are some examples of immature legumes: wax beans, snow peas, edamame, and fresh lima beans.

Immature legumes can be easily incorporated to your meals; they are great in salads and equally delicious when steamed. Mature legumes are harvested from the pod in their fully developed, dried form. Black beans, kidney beans, lentils, and split peas are all mature legumes. Nearly all legumes provide complex carbohydrates, protein, fiber, B vitamins, iron, zinc, magnesium, and potassium.

Health Benefits of Legumes

The glycemic index measures the speed at which carbohydrates from the foods consumed raise the blood sugar during absorption. Foods with high glycemic index values will produce a rapid rise in blood glucose level. This action leads to an increase in secretion of insulin from the pancreas. Type 2 diabetes is developed when there is the combination of chronic elevated blood glucose levels and excessive secretion of insulin. Foods with high fiber content or that are high in complex carbohydrates, like legumes, have a low glycemic index value and thus will not produce the rapid surge in blood sugar levels or the excessive secretion of insulin.

Obesity is a major risk factor for type 2 diabetes. Many studies have shown that the consumption of low-glycemic index foods will increase the sense of fullness, delay the return of hunger, and decrease subsequent food intake as compared with high-glycemic index foods. Including legumes in your diet will help you achieve and maintain a healthy weight. If you are a diabetic, legumes should be your friend at the dinner table. They have insoluble fiber, which gives bulk to stool and promotes bowel regularity. Additionally, it binds cholesterol, thus lowering blood cholesterol level. Therefore, consuming a diet high in legumes will not only help to prevent or reverse type 2 diabetes; it will also protect you against coronary artery disease.

Legumes and whole grains are considered complementary proteins; neither contains all nine essential amino acids, but they form a complete protein when consumed together on the same day. Soybeans, however, are the exception; they provide complete, high-quality protein.

Legumes are easy to use in your meals. They can be added to salads or soups. They can be sautéed, spiced, and served over brown rice. They can be made into dips like hummus, which is a mixture of chickpeas, lemon juice, tahini paste, and garlic. This can be served with pita bread or crackers or as a dip for raw vegetable sticks.

I usually have a wide variety of beans and peas in my pantry. Now if you would like to protect yourself from diseases such as diabetes, heart disease, obesity, and hypertension, you too should fill your pantry with legumes.

Despite the many health benefits from legumes, some people refuse to consume them because of the common side effects. Since legumes are high in fiber, they are not completely digested and this has its own health benefits. However, some people may experience some intestinal discomfort and gas production (flatulence). To reduce the intestinal discomfort, here are some tips:

1. Soak packaged raw legumes for a few hours before cooking. You must also pour off the water you used to soak the legumes.
2. When using canned beans, you should pour off the water and rinse before cooking.

3. If you have not been consuming legumes, then start by introducing a small amount to your meal—two to three tablespoons. This will help your digestive system become used to processing this new food. As the flatulence decreases, you can slowly increase the amount of legumes in your diet.

A diet high in legumes may lower cholesterol, reduce the risk of many cancers, improve blood glucose control in diabetics, help to prevent diabetes, lower blood pressure, prevent and cure constipation, and prevent the formation of diverticulosis and hemorrhoids.

Fiber Content in Beans and Legumes	
Types of Beans and Legumes (1 Cup Cooked)	Grams of Fiber
lentils	16
red kidney beans	16
black beans	15
pinto beans	15
soy nuts (soya beans)	14
adzuki beans (red beans)	13
Anasazi beans	12
chickpeas (garbanzo)	12
pigeon beans	11
fava beans (road beans)	9
lima beans	9
black-eyed peas	8
butter beans	8
edamame (green soybeans)	8
peanuts	3

CHAPTER 8

Fruits and Vegetables: The Super Foods

*T*he word is out. Fruits and vegetables will keep diseases in retreat! Have you noticed people around you either juicing or making smoothies from fruits and vegetables? You may have wondered if the world is getting healthier. Is there real potential to become healthier if you consume more fruits and vegetables?

Taking a look at the diet given in the beginning of human existence, the Bible reveals that fruits and vegetables were an integral part of the original diet given to Adam and Eve. No wonder they and their early descendants enjoyed long life spans! As the world continues to move away from this original diet, we are faced with more diseases that shorten our longevity. Today, scientists are confirming that the consumption of fruits and vegetables will indeed protect against many diseases, such as diabetes, hypertension, heart disease, and cancer.

VEGETABLES

Nutrient-dense green vegetables—leafy greens, cruciferous vegetables, and other green vegetables—are the most important foods to focus on in your diet. In fact, greens are the number-one food you can eat regularly to help improve your health. For maximum health benefits, you should aim to consume five or more servings of vegetables per day. These types of foods are even known to aid in the prevention and reversal of diabetes. Higher green vegetable consumption is associated with lower risk of developing type 2 diabetes, and among diabetics, higher green vegetable intake is associated with lowering HbA1c levels. A recent meta-analysis found that greater leafy green intake was associated with a 14 percent decrease in risk of type 2 diabetes. One study reported that each daily serving of leafy greens produces a 9 percent decrease in the risk of developing diabetes. Kale is known as a powerhouse. It is a nutrient-rich food that is an excellent source of vitamins A, C, and K. It also has a good amount of calcium and supplies folate and potassium. Other noteworthy greens include the following:

- ✓ broccoli
- ✓ collard greens
- ✓ romaine lettuce
- ✓ spinach

Nonstarchy vegetables, like mushrooms, onions, garlic, eggplant, and peppers are essential components of a chronic illness prevention (or reversal) diet. These foods have almost nonexistent effects on blood glucose and are packed with fiber and phytochemicals. They are also very low in calories; therefore, they are excellent for weight loss or maintaining a healthy weight.

FRUITS

Most fruits are naturally low in fat, sodium, and calories, and, as with vegetables, none of them contain cholesterol. They are good sources of many essential nutrients that are underconsumed in our society today, including the following:

- ✓ dietary fiber
- ✓ folate (folic acid)
- ✓ potassium
- ✓ vitamin C

Research shows that healthy potassium consumption in a person's diet may help to maintain healthy blood pressure. Dietary fiber obtained from fruits helps to reduce blood cholesterol levels and may even lower a person's risk of heart disease. It is important to note, however, that although whole or cut fruits are great sources of dietary fiber, *fruit juices* may contain little or no fiber at all.

Fruits are also great sources of vitamin C, which is important for the growth and repair of all body tissues. It also helps heal cuts and wounds and keeps teeth and gums healthy. Folate (folic acid) helps the body form red blood cells. Women of childbearing age who may become pregnant should consume adequate folate from foods such as citrus fruits (oranges, limes, grapefruits, berries, papaya, and cantaloupe). This reduces the risk of neural tube defects, spina bifida, and anencephaly during fetal development.

How and How Much to Consume?

You will now agree with me that fruits and vegetables are important for a balanced and healthy diet; in fact, it is recommended that half of your plate be filled with fruits and vegetables. Remember that different fruits and vegetables contain unique vitamins, minerals, and phytonutrients, so the consumption of a variety of fruits and vegetables is important. When you consume a variety of types and colors of fruits and vegetables, you will give your body a mix of nutrients it needs to maintain good health. You should try to incorporate dark leafy greens and brightly colored red, yellow, and orange vegetables and fruits to your diet.

It is relatively easy to find fruits and vegetables of different colors; however, consuming an adequate amount per day may be more difficult. I usually recommend to my patients that they should consume eight to ten servings of fruits and vegetables a day. This they find alarming and more of a challenge to do. However, if you make it a habit to include fruits and vegetables with each meal or if you create recipes in which fruits and vegetables are the main ingredients, then it becomes easier to obtain the required daily amounts.

For maximum benefit, it is best to consume your vegetables raw (salads) or slightly steamed. Overcooking the vegetables will lead to loss of essential nutrients, such as vitamins and minerals. Fruits should be consumed whole; when the juice is extracted, most of the fiber will be lost. As mentioned before, fiber is of utmost importance to maintaining good health. If you wish to liquefy your fruits, then smoothies are better than juice extraction. With the smoothie, the fiber is also consumed.

BENEFITS ON GENERAL HEALTH

Not long ago the book *The Blue Zone* published reports on a few regions in the world where the populations were enjoying health and living longer than one hundred years. The author of the book reveals that the people who live in these *blue zones* had something in common; they were mostly vegetarians. Among a few other common factors, these centurions had a diet that was mostly plant-based.

BENEFITS ON CARDIOVASCULAR HEALTH

Most fruits and vegetables are naturally low in fats and calories but have a high content of potassium. These properties promote low blood pressure and low risk of coronary artery disease. In a study conducted at the Harvard School of Public Health, Dr. K. J. Joshipura and his colleagues reported that Americans consuming the most fruits and vegetables were at a 20 percent lower risk of developing coronary artery disease than those consuming hardly any fruits and vegetables. This study also revealed that risk of stroke was reduced by 31 percent in those participants who consumed more fruits and vegetables.

BLOOD PRESSURE

While sodium will increase blood pressure, potassium has the reverse effect. Fruits and vegetables have a high content of dietary potassium, which has a positive effect on keeping the blood pressure low. The *Dietary Approaches to Stop Hypertension* (DASH) study examined the effect on blood pressure of a diet that was rich in fruits, vegetables, and low-fat dairy products and that restricted the amount of saturated and total fat. The researchers found that people with high blood pressure who followed this diet reduced their systolic blood pressure (the upper number of a blood pressure reading) by about 11 mmHg and their diastolic blood pressure (the lower number) by almost 6 mmHg—as much as medications can achieve. The DASH method is now being recommended to patients with high blood pressure as a therapeutic approach to control hypertension.

CANCER

Scientists have discovered that each fruit and vegetable provides unique vitamins, minerals, and phytochemicals; therefore, different fruits and vegetables protect against different diseases. In a study conducted by the Harvard Medical School, it was reported that the consumption of cruciferous vegetables such as broccoli, cauliflower, kale, brussels sprouts, and cabbage reduces the risk of colon cancer.

DIABETES

As mentioned before, most fruits and vegetables are high in fiber and low in calories. They are usually low-glycemic index foods, which means that during digestion, there is a slow and steady absorption of glucose into the bloodstream. The consumption of fruits and vegetables instead of foods such as rice and potatoes will lead to better blood sugar control or will prevent or reverse type 2 diabetes. Diabetics should include green leafy and nonstarchy vegetables in their diet. Fruits, such as berries, cantaloupes, pears, kiwis, tomatoes, and plums, are great for diabetics.

Glycemic Index and Load Table		
Food Type	**GI**	**GL**
glucose	100	10
white potato	85	26
watermelon	72	4
white rice	72	16
white bread	70	10
cantaloupe	65	4
sweet potato	61	17
pineapple	59	7
wild rice	57	16
honey	55	10
maple syrup	54	10
kiwi	53	6
mango	51	8
ripe banana	51	13
brown rice	50	16
whole wheat bread	49	9
grapes	46	8
peach	42	5
white pasta	41	26
strawberry/blueberry	40	1
apple	38	6
pear	38	4
whole wheat pasta	38	17
chickpeas / kidney beans	28	8
cashew nuts	25	3
cherries	22	3
agave	19	2
cauliflower	15	2
eggplant	15	2
lettuce, spinach	15	1
soybeans	18	1
tomato, zucchini	15	2
broccoli, mushroom	10	4
cabbage	10	2
kale	2	3

Diabetic patients should choose foods with very low glycemic index in order to improve their health or reverse their disease

Obesity

It is a well-known fact that consuming the ideal foods in the right portion is paramount for maintaining a healthy weight. Since fiber-rich fruits and vegetables gives bulk to the diet, the sensation of fullness is achieved early and digestion is usually slow; therefore, you will feel full longer. Since the hunger is suppressed, there will be a longer fasting period between meals and the need to snack will be decreased. As you consume fewer calories and less frequently, you will notice the pounds disappearing without the need to starve yourself. You can surely have more on your plate and yet weigh less if you consume the right foods.

Some people will purchase lots of fruits and vegetables and then allow these precious foods to go bad in the refrigerator. Of course, to ensure that you include these foods in your diet, you need to have them at hand. If you find that you are not using them enough, make them the start of your main dish (salad, vegetable soup) or put them all together in one dish, hot or cold. Just be creative! A patient once told me that he made a delicious "garbage soup." I was left startled, not knowing what he meant. I questioned him. He replied, "Yes, doc, I just throw into a pot all the vegetables I had in my refrigerator." Smart man indeed. You too can make your garbage soup and you will no longer have spoilage of super fruits and vegetables.

When you place fruits and vegetables as the centerpiece on your dinner table, you will not only receive all the amazing health benefits these foods provide; you will keep chronic diseases in retreat.

CHAPTER 9

Meats: Red and Processed—Are They Safe?

A report by the US Department of Agriculture revealed that the average American consumed 74 pounds of red meat and 55 pounds of poultry in 2012. It projected that these numbers would significantly increase in 2016. Recently, there has been a high alert on the consumption of processed meats and the possible health dangers posed. Researchers were able to conclude that the consumption of processed meat was directly linked to an increased risk of diseases, such as cancer and coronary heart disease. Do you consume processed meats? Would you like to learn about the health risks of eating processed meats? In the *Journal of the American Medical Association*, published online July 10, 2013, it was reported that, dietary risk factor is the leading cause of chronic diseases and death in the United States and in other parts of the world. Over the next several weeks, the high alert on health and the consumption of processed meats made major news headlines. It is almost certain that this information has generated many questions to which many are seeking answers. One might wonder whether the problem is the meat or the processing of it. Or could it be both?

Let's begin with defining processed meats. These are meats preserved using the following methods: curing, salting, smoking, or adding chemicals, such as sodium nitrite. Some examples of processed meats include bacon, ham, salami, hot dogs, corned beef, bologna, sausage, and beef jerky, just to name a few.

Processed meats have a long shelf life. Adding chemicals, such as nitrites, or any nitrous compounds will preserve the red or pink color of the meat and will improve flavor by suppressing fat oxidation. Processing the meat will also prevent the growth of bacteria, thus reducing the risk of food poisoning.

Researchers now believe that the consumption of meats preserved with nitrites or nitrous compounds increases the risk for developing cancer, especially cancer of the stomach and colon.

Other harmful chemicals, such as polycyclic aromatic hydrocarbons, are formed during the smoking of meat. These chemicals are also produced during barbecuing, grilling, and roasting. These harmful compounds are transferred from wood, coal, or hot surfaces into the air before accumulating on the surface of the meat products. Studies have shown that these polycyclic aromatic hydrocarbons are also cancer-causing agents.

Salting of meat, an old practice, is also dangerous for one's health. A diet high in sodium increases the risk of hypertension, which in turn increases the risk of heart disease and death.

Researchers at Harvard Medical School conducted a study that included 120,000 candidates and proved that a diet high in red meat can shorten the life expectancy by increasing one's risk of death from cancer and heart-related problems. The researchers analyzed data from 37,698 men between 1986 and 2008 and 83,644 women between 1980 and 2008.

The study revealed that adding an extra portion of unprocessed red meat to someone's daily diet increases the risk of death from any cause by 13 percent, fatal cardiovascular disease by 18 percent, and cancer mortality by 10 percent. The figures recorded for those who consumed processed meat were even higher—20 percent for the overall mortality rate, 21 percent for deaths from heart-related diseases, and 16 percent for cancer mortality.

A study published in the *Archives of Internal Medicine* cited that a high intake of processed and unprocessed red meat is associated with a significantly elevated risk of cardiovascular disease and cancer mortality. Moreover, there is a relatively greater risk with the consumption of processed meat.

The researchers suggested that the saturated fat from red meat may be the main factor that causes an increased risk for heart-related diseases and the sodium used in processed meat may increase the risk of developing cardiovascular diseases through its effect on blood pressure.

It is therefore safe to conclude that avoiding both processed and unprocessed meat will decrease your risk of dying early from some cancers and cardiovascular diseases.

You may wonder how you will obtain enough protein if you should remove red meat from your diet. The truth of the matter is contrary to what most people believe; you do not need a large amount of protein in your diet to be in good health. On average, people only need about 60 grams of protein daily; only about 25 to 30 percent of your daily caloric intake should be from protein. In other words, a quarter of the food on your plate at mealtime should be protein. Isn't that good news? Even when you remove all animal products from your diet, there is nothing to fear; you will find enough protein in fruits, vegetables, nuts, grains, and seeds. You will find tables in this chapter listing the protein content in certain foods.

Protein Content in Whole Grains	
Types Of Whole Grains (1 Cup Cooked)	**Grams of Protein**
rye	25
sorghum	22
spelt	11
amaranth	9
farro	8
quinoa	8
wheat	7
whole wheat pasta	7
wild rice	7
buckwheat	6
bulgur	6
millet	6
oats	6
brown rice	5
corn kernel	5
barley	4
whole wheat bread	4
white bread	4

Protein Content in Beans and Legumes

Types of Beans and Legumes (1 Cup Cooked)	Grams of Protein
soy nuts (soya beans)	68
lentils	18
edamame	17
red kidney beans	16
adzuki beans (red beans)	15
black beans	15
chickpeas (garbanzo beans)	15
pinto beans	15
Anasazi beans	14
fava beans	13
lima beans	12
pigeon beans	11
black-eyed peas	5
butter beans	5
peanuts	5

The usual recommended daily amount of protein is 0.8mg/kg; the average person with a weight of 75 kg will have a need of 60 mg daily.

CHAPTER 10

Physical Exercise Is Medicine

*I*t is not a secret that regular physical exercise is now seen as an important predictor of good health and longevity. In fact, when prescribing an action plan that is geared toward good health and disease prevention, I know physical exercise goes hand in hand with a healthy diet. Researchers have suggested that inactivity might even be more detrimental to our health than smoking. This is remarkable!

It is believed that less than 25 percent of Americans receive regular physical activity daily; hence, the incidence of obesity and diseases, such as diabetes, hypertension, heart disease, and cancer, are on the rise. The benefits of physical exercise extend far beyond weight management. Research has also shown that regular physical exercise can help reduce one's risk of several diseases and health conditions and improve overall quality of life.

Many studies have shown a direct relationship between mortality and inactivity. Published in the *Journal of the American Medical Association*, December 5, 2007, was a report that people who get regular physical exercise can reduce their chances of health-related illnesses by 50 to 73 percent while decreasing the mortality rate. The risk of cancer mortality is reduced to less than 50 percent in those receiving moderate to vigorous physical exercise for at least thirty minutes daily.

The *Physical Activity Guidelines* for Americans recommends that all adults get at least thirty minutes of moderate physical exercise daily for six days a week. You may wonder what moderate exercise is. Some experts believe that moderate exercise will cause you to break a sweat. You could also exercise to achieve at least 75 percent of your maximum heart rate. To find know that, just subtract your age from 220; the number remaining is the maximum heart rate. Now the goal is to achieve 75 percent of that number. Let's say that you are twenty years old. Your maximum heart rate would be 200, but the desired heart rate to achieve would be 75 percent of 200, which would be 150.

The health literature reveals that as many as one in twelve of all deaths per year is a consequence of lack of physical activity. Would you believe that exercise is then protective against many health conditions? Let's look at a few health benefits that you should expect from regular physical exercise:

- reduces the risk of high blood pressure
- reduces the risk of heart disease
- reduces the risk of diabetes
- improves mood and decreases the risk of depression and anxiety
- builds stronger bones and prevents fractures
- improves immunity
- helps with weight loss
- maintains muscle mass
- improves glucose tolerance and insulin sensitivity
- improves the blood lipid profile by decreasing triglycerides and increasing the good cholesterol (HDL)
- increases energy and physical endurance

I recommend that you start with a goal. You must define what you hope to achieve, which could be more energy, muscle strengthening, a healthier weight, better blood pressure, or diabetes control. Here are some great tips to follow:

START SLOW

You could begin by walking three to four times weekly for ten to fifteen minutes; this time could be increased as you become more comfortable. Remember to aim for a minimum of thirty minutes daily for at least six days weekly. If your goal is to lose weight, then obtaining at least sixty minutes of moderate physical exercise daily is recommended. Remember, there are more health benefits as you increase the intensity and duration of physical exercise, but, like with anything else, moderation is the key. Too much of a good thing may be detrimental to your health.

CHOOSE AN ACTIVITY THAT YOU ENJOY

For most people, walking is the simplest form of exercise they can do, but if you are young and more active, then activities such as biking, jogging, and swimming are great. Golfing, gardening, mowing the lawn, and dancing are also excellent forms of physical exercise. Whenever possible, climb the stairs instead of taking the elevator or escalator and don't forget to park farther away and walk. The most important thing to remember is to remain physically active. It is also good to have an exercise partner, someone who will encourage you, make it fun, and hold you accountable.

Many times, as I counsel my patients, the question of the best time to exercise is a part of that conversation, but is there really a best time? Exercise is medicine and should be seen as a priority. Once this is understood, the time for exercise should not be a problem. I like to exercise early in the morning when I am more energized. I also realize that if I do not exercise at the beginning of the day, I will have a problem finding enough time to exercise. Stay focused, keep your eyes on the goals that you initially set for yourself, and reward yourself when you achieve those goals.

Everyone can participate in some form of physical activity regardless of age or physical challenges. If you are elderly and have not been physically active, speak with your health care provider before you begin exercising. There are people with diseases, such as arthritis, high blood pressure, and lung or heart disease who may be hesitant to participate in any form of physical activity. If you are such a person, then discuss your plans with your health care provider and ask for medical clearance. Many health care providers now understand the therapeutic role that regular physical exercise plays not only in disease prevention but also in the actual treatment of many chronic diseases, such as diabetes, hypertension, osteoporosis, and heart disease. Therefore, many physicians are now prescribing exercise in similar manner as we do medicines.

I will share a story with you to emphasize the health benefit of exercise. An elderly man presented to my office with difficulty breathing, irregular heart rate, depression, obesity, and high blood pressure; he was obviously very ill. This patient had been in and out of the hospital with heart failure and arrhythmia about eleven times in less than one year. After a thorough assessment, I formulated a treatment plan with his consent. Included in his care plan was a regimen of regular physical exercise. I will never forget what this patient told me when I revealed to him the treatment plan. He said, "Doc, I can only get from my bed to the chair." Needless to say, I encouraged him and got him enrolled in my lifestyle program. He started a therapeutic nutritional plan along with daily physical exercise. The patient slowly started to become more active. Initially he needed a walker for mobility, then he graduated from the walker to a cane. Now, he is able to walk independently without support. You may be wondering about his general health. His story is quite exciting! He lost weight, his heart function improved, he became happier, his depression was resolved, and most important, he no longer needs inpatient care. This patient is only one of my many who have dramatically altered their health destinies using exercise in combination with other therapeutic lifestyle modifications. Staying physically active will help you prevent, improve, or reverse many chronic diseases as you continue on your journey to a healthier, happier, and more abundant life.

CHAPTER 11

The Program Made Simple

*N*ow that you have read the preceding chapters and have seen that there is indeed hope beyond those medications for whatever disease you may have, I am sure that you are excited and ready to start a healthy lifestyle-change program. So how does it work?

The Fourteen Days to Amazing Health program is designed to educate, inspire, and empower you to use simple lifestyle choices that are essential in preventing or reversing chronic diseases, such as diabetes, hypertension, cardiovascular diseases, obesity, chronic pain, and even some cancers.

THE ESSENTIALS OF THE PROGRAM

1. The very first thing to do as you begin the program is to assess your overall health.
2. Establish your goals. What do you want to change? Would you like to decrease the number of medications you are currently taking? Is your goal to obtain a healthier weight? Or would you like to lower your blood pressure or reverse diabetes?
3. Make a visit with your health care provider. Discuss your plans to change your lifestyle and obtain complete laboratory tests (cholesterol level, blood sugar level, HbA1c, and so on).

4. Commit yourself to the fourteen-day meal plan and recipes laid out for you in this book.

5. Consume whole-grain plant-based foods during the fourteen days and beyond.

6. Avoid the consumption of animal-based foods.

7. Limit the intake of vegetable oils, nut butter, sugar, and salt.

8. Eliminate sodas, coffee, and alcohol and increase your intake of water.

9. Make breakfast your most important meal of the day, and make dinner your lightest meal.

10. Avoid eating late at night. (I strongly recommended no meals after five in the evening.)

11. Exercise for at least thirty to sixty minutes daily.

12. Get seven to eight hours of sleep per night.

13. Spend ten to fifteen minutes per day enjoying the sunlight.

14. Meditate for twenty to thirty minutes daily. A suggested text from the Bible is given for you to read during your time of meditation.

15. Maintain a positive attitude and be grateful.

16. Read and incorporate the daily health facts given to reinforce evidence-based medicine in relationship to the suggested lifestyle changes.

17. Document your progress.

Don't be alarmed by the long list. The plan is truly simple. The *Get Healthy with Dr. Cooper* program is not designed only to ensure physical health but also for you to enjoy "whole person health," which includes mental, social, and spiritual well-being. This is a holistic approach to a happier, healthier, and more fulfilled life.

Assess Your Health Status

How Healthy Are You?

Instructions—For each health indicator, check the box in the column that best describes you. Write the score for that column in the score column on the right.

Health Indicators	Column A 0	Column B 5	Column C 10	Score
1. Disease—Do you have high blood pressure?	Yes, uncontrolled	Yes, controlled	No	_____
2. Disease—Do you have diabetes?	Yes, uncontrolled	Yes, controlled	No	_____
3. Disease—Do you have heart disease?	Yes, uncontrolled	Yes, controlled	No	_____
4. Body weight—What is your body mass index? (BMI chart in week 5)	BMI 30+	BMI 25–29.9	BMI <25	_____
5. Blood pressure—What is your blood pressure?	140/90+	120/80–139/89	<120/80	_____
6. Physical activity—Do you engage in at least 30 minutes daily of moderate or vigorous exercise?	No regular physical exercise	2–3 days per week	5–7 days per week	_____
7. Fruits and vegetables—How many servings daily do you consume? (1 serving = 1 medium fruit, 1/2 cup cooked vegetables, 1 cup raw vegetables)	0–3	4–5	6–9	_____
8. Whole grain—How many servings per day do you consume? (1 serving = 1 slice whole wheat bread, 2/3 cup brown rice, oatmeal, quinoa, or dry cereal)	<1/day	1–2 servings/day	3+ servings/day	_____

9. Legumes—How many servings of legumes do you have per day? (1 serving = 1/2 cup cooked beans, peas, or lentils)	<1 servings per day	1–2 servings per day	3 or more servings per day	_____
10. Nuts and seeds—How many servings do you have per week? (1 serving = 1 ounce nuts or seeds, 2 tablespoons of nut butter)	0–2 servings per week	2–4 servings per week	5 or more servings per week	_____
11. Red and processed meats—How many servings of meat do you have per day? (egg, beef, ham, sausage, salami; (1 serving = 3 ounces)	>3 servings per day	1–2 servings per day	<1 serving per day	_____
12. Snack foods—How many times per week do you consume candy bars, chips, fries, and sodas?	>7 times per week	2–6 times per week	<1 per week	_____
13. Water—How many cups of water do you drink daily?	<5 cups per day	6–7 cups per day	8 or more cups per day	_____
14. Breakfast—Do you have breakfast regularly?	Seldom	Sometimes	Daily	_____
15. Sleep—What is the average amount of hours you sleep per day?	<5 hours per day	<7 hours per day	7–9 hours per day	_____
16. Sugar—What is your blood sugar level, if known?	126+	100–125	<100	_____
17. Blood cholesterol—What is your LDL cholesterol level, if known?	160+	130–159	<130	_____
18. Smoking status—Indicate your present status.	Current smoker	Ex-smoker	Nonsmoker	
19. Social relationships—Indicate your current status.	Have no social or family support / rarely connect	Some family and social support / connect occasionally	Strong family and social support / frequently connect	_____
20. Happiness—How happy are you?	Not happy, often sad or depressed	Somewhat happy / seldom sad	Very happy and satisfied with life	_____

21. Time outdoors—How much time do you spend outdoors?	<10 min. per day	10–30 min. per day	30 or more min. per day	_____
22. Hope and the future— What is your outlook on the future?	Pessimistic	Somewhat optimistic	Very optimistic	_____
23. Spiritual connection / meditation—Indicate your current status.	No spiritual or religious belief. I do not meditate.	I am learning about spiritual values / meditate often.	I have faith and engage regularly with people of the same faith. / I meditate regularly.	_____

Total lifestyle score _____

0–60 very high risk	65–100 moderate risk	105–150 average risk	155–200 good	205–300 excellent

Body Mass Index Chart

Height (Ft/Ins)	Normal						Overweight					Obese					
																	Weight in pounds
4'10"	91	96	100	105	110	115	119	124	129	134	138	143	148	153	158	162	167
4'11"	94	99	104	109	114	119	124	128	133	138	143	148	153	158	163	168	173
5'	97	102	107	112	118	123	128	133	138	143	148	153	158	163	168	174	179
5'1"	100	106	111	116	122	127	132	137	143	148	153	158	164	169	174	180	185
5'2"	104	109	115	120	126	131	136	142	147	153	158	164	169	175	180	186	191
5'3"	107	113	118	124	130	135	141	146	152	158	163	169	175	180	186	191	197
5'4"	110	116	122	128	134	140	145	151	157	163	169	174	180	186	192	197	204
5'5"	114	120	126	132	138	144	150	156	162	168	174	180	186	192	198	204	210
5'6"	118	124	130	136	142	148	155	161	167	173	179	186	192	198	204	210	216
5'7"	121	127	134	140	146	153	159	166	172	178	185	191	198	204	211	217	223
5'8"	125	131	138	144	151	158	164	171	177	184	190	197	203	210	216	223	230
5'9"	128	135	142	149	155	162	169	176	182	189	196	203	209	216	223	230	236
5'10"	132	139	146	153	160	167	174	181	188	195	202	209	216	222	229	236	243
5'11"	136	143	150	157	165	172	179	186	193	200	208	215	222	229	236	243	250
6'	140	147	154	162	169	177	184	191	199	206	213	221	228	235	242	250	258
6'1"	144	151	159	166	174	182	189	197	204	212	219	227	235	242	250	257	265
6'2"	148	155	163	171	179	186	194	202	210	218	225	233	241	249	256	264	272
6'3"	152	160	168	176	184	192	200	208	216	224	232	240	248	256	264	272	279
6'4"	156	164	172	180	189	197	205	213	221	230	238	246	254	263	271	279	287
BMI	19	20	21	22	23	24	25	26	27	28	29	30	31	32	33	34	35

Use this chart to determine your BMI, and use this number to answer the questions on the previous pages.

Personal Goals

Check or select all the changes you wish to implement that will promote better personal health.

- ☐ achieve and maintain a healthier weight
- ☐ improve or reverse diabetes
- ☐ improve or reverse hypertension
- ☐ improve overall health
- ☐ reduce medications
- ☐ improve physical endurance
- ☐ eat at least eight servings of fruits and vegetables daily
- ☐ eat a least five servings of whole grains weekly
- ☐ reduce the consumption of processed or refined foods
- ☐ increase the intake of nuts and seeds
- ☐ get at least thirty minutes of physical exercise daily, a minimum of six days weekly
- ☐ get seven to eight hours of timely rest per night
- ☐ spend more time with family and friends
- ☐ have devotional exercise or meditation at least twenty to thirty minutes per day
- ☐ to live disease free for life

My Commitment

It is my deepest desire to implement the changes listed above, as I embrace the information outlined in this book.

My signature

PART 2

Living the Amazing Health Plan

CHAPTER 12

Fourteen Days Program Details

DAY 1

Breakfast
- cashew oats waffle (1 serving with strawberry dressing)
- nondairy milk (1 cup)
- fruits (one cup cantaloupe)

Lunch
- black bean (1/2 cup)
- quinoa salad* (1/2 cup)
- apple (1 medium)

Dinner
- garden minestrone soup* (2 cups)
- raw vegetables salad (abundant)
- avocado salad dressing* (2 tablespoons)
- fresh fruit (1 kiwi)

Exercise
Level 1
- Warm up. Start with a five-minute walk at a moderate pace.
- Walk for sixty seconds at a revved-up pace.
- Walk for thirty seconds at a moderate pace.
- Repeat ten times.

- Do calf raises, three sets, twelve to fifteen repetitions.
- Cool down. End with a five-minute walk at an easy pace.

Level 2:
- Warm up. Start with a five-minute walk at a moderate pace.
- Walk for sixty seconds at a revved-up pace.
- Walk for thirty seconds at a moderate pace.
- Repeat twelve times.
- Do standing leg curls, three sets, twelve to fifteen repetitions.
- Cool down. End with a five-minute walk at an easy pace.

Level 3
- Warm up. Start with a five-minute walk at a moderate pace.
- Walk for sixty seconds at a revved-up pace.
- Walk for thirty seconds at a moderate pace.
- Repeat fifteen times.
- Do side hip raises, three sets, fifteen to twenty repetitions.
- Cool down. End with a five-minute walk at an easy pace.

Meditation
- Reflect on the goals that you have set for yourself. Meditate on the reason or reasons why you would like to make a change in lifestyle. Seek help from a higher power; take time to meditate, practice yoga, or pray daily.

Health Facts—Healing with Grains
- Research has confirmed that the consumption of at least five servings of whole grains daily in combination with cruciferous vegetables and folic acid may reduce the risk of colon cancer.
- Whole grains are great sources of complex carbohydrates and provide essential nutrients, such as vitamin E, thiamine, iron, and magnesium, all of which are important for cell function.

---

* indicate that recipes are in the recipes section of the book.

- Processed grains, such as white flour or white rice, contain 75 to 80 percent less fiber and phytochemicals than whole grains. Processed grains shorten your life span. For this reason, I recommend that you avoid all processed grains while you are on this program.
- Dietary fiber gives bulk to stool; this increases bowel regularity, prevents constipation, and lowers the risk of diverticulosis.
- Dietary fiber lowers cholesterol and thus decreases the risk of cardiovascular disease. It stabilizes blood glucose and thus could improve, prevent, or reverse diabetes.
- The US Department of Agriculture recommends that at least half of all grains in the diet be whole grains.
- Read the chapter in the book on whole grains or watch the *Get Healthy with Dr. Cooper* DVD series (www.cooperwellnesscenter.com).

Document

Keep a record of your weight, blood pressure, and blood sugar (if you have diabetes).

Weight_____BP_____BS_____

Daily Lesson

You have a choice in your health destiny.

DAY 2

Breakfast
- old-fashioned oats with cinnamon* (1 cup)
- grapefruit (half)
- flaxseed (1 tablespoon mixed in the oats)

Lunch

- walnut balls* (3)
- whole wheat pasta (1 cup)
- fresh green vegetable salad (abundant)
- Caesar salad dressing (2 tablespoons)
- pear (1 medium)

Dinner
- white bean kale soup* (2 cups)
- steamed asparagus with Caesar salad dressings*
- cantaloupe (1 cup)

Exercise
Level 1
- Warm up. Start with a five-minute walk at a moderate pace.
- Walk for sixty seconds at a revved-up pace.
- Walk for thirty seconds at a moderate pace.
- Repeat fifteen times.
- Do side hip raises, three sets, fifteen to twenty repetitions.
- Cool down. End with a five-minute walk at an easy pace.

Level 2
- Warm up. Start with a seven-minute walk at a moderate pace.
- Do side-to-side squat jump, three sets, ten to fifteen repetitions.
- Do in-place forward lunges, three sets, twelve to fifteen reps.
- Do bicep curls, three sets, eight to twelve repetitions.

- Do single leg lifts, three sets, twelve to fifteen repetitions.
- Cool down. End with seven-minute walk at an easy pace.

Level 3
- Warm up. Start with a seven-minute walk at a moderate pace.
- Do burpee jacks, three sets, thirty seconds.
- Do kettlebell squats, three sets, twelve to fifteen repetitions.
- Do bridges, three sets, twelve to fifteen repetitions.
- Do planks, three sets, fifteen seconds.
- Cool down. End with a seven-minute walk at an easy pace.

Meditation
- Meditate on someone who has had a positive influence in your life. Read 3 John 1:2 (KJV): "Beloved, I wish above all things that thou mayest prosper and be in health, even as thy soul prospereth"

Health Facts—Inactivity Will Sabotage Your Health.
- Researchers now state that inactivity is slightly more harmful to your health than smoking. It is proven that exercise is one of the most important predictors of longevity, yet only about 20 percent of all Americans receive regular physical activity daily. Could this be the reason for the obesity and diabetes crises in the United States?
- A study reported in the *Journal of the American Medical Association* noted the risk of death was 50 to 73 percent less in those who are engaged in regular exercise when compared to inactive persons. Regular physical exercise decreases the risk of colon cancer as well as breast cancer.
- The *Physical Activity Guidelines* recommend two and a half hours of physical exercise weekly for all Americans.
- There should not be any excuses for not obtaining physical exercise. In this book, I have laid out three levels of exercises that you may engage in. If you are a beginner, level one is designed with you in mind. If you are in a wheelchair, then exercise the

upper body. If you use a cane or a walker, then walk with support or get active by doing the chair exercises.

- As you may have discovered by now, exercise is medicine. There are several health benefits that you will receive from regular physical exercise (read the chapter on exercise), but in order to reach your full health potential, you must follow through.

- In 1905, a Christian author, E. G. White wrote, "All who can possibly do so ought to walk in the open air every day, summer, and winter. A walk even in winter would be more beneficial to health than all the medicines the doctors may prescribe."

- Read the chapter on exercise in this book or watch the *Get Healthy with Dr. Cooper* DVD series (visit www.cooperwellnesscenter.com).

Document

Keep track of weight _____ BP_____BS_____.

Daily Lesson

- What are you waiting for? Invest in your health by simply walking briskly daily and reap the rewards later with a longer and happier life.

Day 3

Breakfast

- bean spread* (1/4 cup)
- whole wheat bread (1 slice)
- chopped tomato and lettuce (abundant)
- fruit (6 strawberries)

Lunch

- tabbouleh* (2 cups)
- pita bread (1 serving)
- fruit (melon)

Dinner

- lentil soup (1 cup)
- green leafy vegetables (abundant)
- cashew nuts (8 whole nuts)

Exercise

Level 1

- Warm up: Start with a five-minute walk at a moderate pace.
- Walk for sixty seconds at a revved-up pace.
- Walk for thirty seconds at a moderate pace.
- Repeat ten times.
- Do calf raises, three sets, twelve to fifteen repetitions.
- Cool down. End with five-minute walk at an easy pace.

Level 2

- Warm up. Start with a five-minute walk at a moderate pace.
- Walk for sixty seconds at a revved-up pace.
- Walk for thirty seconds at a moderate pace.
- Repeat twelve times.

- Do standing leg curls, three sets, twelve to fifteen repetitions.
- Cool down. End with a five-minute walk at an easy pace.

Level 3

- Warm up. Start with a five-minute walk at a moderate pace.
- Walk for sixty seconds at a revved-up pace.
- Walk for thirty seconds at a moderate pace.
- Repeat fifteen times.
- Do side hip raises, three sets, fifteen to twenty repetitions.
- Cool down. End with a five-minute walk at an easy pace.

Meditation

- Meditate on the change you have embarked on and the positive influence that change will have on your life and health in general. Learn about Daniel's plan. Read Daniel 1:12–15.

Health Facts—Water a Natural Remedy

- The body is 70 percent water; therefore, in order to maintain good health, keeping the body well hydrated is important. Lack of adequate intake of water may cause certain health conditions, such as headache, tiredness or fatigue, confusion, gallstones, kidney stones, constipation, blood clots, and urinary tract infection.
- Researchers from the University of Loma Linda in California reported that the consumption of five or more glasses of water a day can significantly decrease your risk of heart attack by 50 percent. Dr. Jacqueline Chen from the University of Loma Linda states, "Not drinking enough water can be as harmful to your health as smoking."
- Eighty percent of people living in America as well as in other parts of the world are chronically dehydrated; they consume less than the required amount of water per day. This increases the risk of acquiring many diseases, including venous blood clots in addition to the others previously mentioned.

- Water is vital to health. The amount that you need is dependent on many factors, including your health, where you live, and how active you are. If you live in a hot climate or if you work outdoors, then you need to drink more water than those who live in or work in the cooler environments or those who are being treated for heart or kidney failure. However, in general, eight eight-ounce glasses of water daily is the usual recommended amount.
- The adequate consumption of water daily will improve mood, enhance physical endurance, treat headaches, help with weight loss, help to treat or prevent kidney stones, and help to treat or prevent constipation.
- The consumption of other fluids, such as tea, coffee, alcohol, or concentrated fruit drinks, instead of water will increase the risk of heart attack by 46 percent (Jacqueline Chen, Loma Linda University).
- Watch "The Fluid That Heals" from the *Get Healthy with Dr. Cooper* DVD series.

Document

- Log your progress: weight _____ BP _____ BS _____.

Daily Lesson

- If you want to achieve amazing health, then make water your preferred drink. Strive to drink at least eight cups daily.

Day 4

Breakfast
- all-bran cereal (1 serving)
- nondairy milk (1 cup)
- fruit salad (1 cup)
- flaxseed (2 tablespoons)

Lunch
- baked sweet potato (1 medium)
- bean chili (1/2 cup)
- leafy greens (abundant)

Dinner
- Indian lentil soup (2 cups)
- green vegetable salad (abundant)
- avocado salad dressing (2 tablespoons)
- walnuts (1 ounce)

Exercise
Level 1
- Warm up. Start with a seven-minute walk at a moderate pace.
- Run in place, three sets, thirty seconds.
- Do air squats, three sets, twelve to fifteen repetitions.
- Do wall push-ups, three sets, eight to twelve repetitions.
- Do crunches, three sets, twelve to fifteen repetitions.
- Cool down. End with a seven-minute walk at an easy pace.

Level 2
- Warm up. Start with a seven-minute walk at a moderate pace.
- Do side-to-side squats, three sets, ten to fifteen repetitions.
- Do in-place forward lunges, three sets, twelve to fifteen repetitions.

- Do bicep curls, three sets, eight to twelve repetitions.
- Do single leg lifts, three sets, twelve to fifteen repetitions.
- Cool down. End with a seven-minute walk at an easy pace.

Level 3

- Warm up. Start with a seven-minute walk at a moderate pace.
- Do burpee jacks, three sets, thirty seconds.
- Do kettlebell squats, three sets, twelve to fifteen repetitions.
- Do bridges, three sets, twelve to fifteen repetitions.
- Do planks, three sets, fifteen seconds.
- Cool down. End with a seven-minute walk at an easy pace.

Meditation

- Meditate on ways to be joyful and happy. List ten things for which you are grateful and the reasons why. Read and memorize Proverbs 17:22 (NIV): "A cheerful heart is good medicine, but a crushed spirit dries up the bones."

Health Facts—Healing with the Sun

- Exposure to sunlight is the main source of vitamin D; however, the health benefits of vitamin D extend far beyond bone health. According to the University of California in San Diego, a study of people living in 177 countries revealed a link between low vitamin D levels and risk of colorectal and breast cancer. The study also revealed that breast and colorectal cancer could be prevented with sufficient exposure to sunlight. This prevention is best achieved with a combination of diet, supplements, and short intervals—ten to fifteen minutes a day—in the sun.
- The Food and Drug Administration (FDA) recommends 1,000 IUs of vitamin D daily, the equivalent of ten to fifteen minutes of sun exposure.
- Vitamin D is a prohormone. It acts as a gene modulator, and therefore adequate levels of vitamin D can prevent gene mutation. Vitamin D can turn off the genes that cause diseases,

including cancer; however, inadequate amounts may lead to several diseases, such as diabetes, osteoporosis, osteomalacia (weak bone with much bone pain), rickets, multiple sclerosis, heart disease, cognitive impairment, cancer, and death.

- Regular exposure to natural sunlight enhances the production of serotonin in the body. Serotonin enhances mood and helps to keep you mentally alert.
- Seasonal affective disorder (SAD) is a type of depression seen in regions where there are long winter months; this limited exposure to sunlight leads to decreased levels of vitamin D and serotonin.
- When the skin is exposed to sunlight, nitric oxide is produced; this substance then lowers blood pressure, which reduces the risk of cardiovascular diseases.
- Watch "The Sunshine Vitamin" from the *Get Healthy with Dr. Cooper* DVD series.

Document
- Track your progress: weight _____ BP_____BS_____.

Daily Lesson

- Smile more today and put some sunlight in the lives of others; better yet, take a short walk in the outdoors today.
- This journey is not a sprint but a marathon; keep focused on your goal. Many have used this program and have been successful. You also are on a journey to succeed.

DAY 5

Breakfast
- cold whole-grain cereal (1 cup)
- berries (1/4 cup)
- walnuts (1 ounce)
- sunflower seeds (2 tablespoons)

Lunch
- chickpea curry* (1/2 cup)
- brown rice (2/3 cup)
- steamed broccoli and cauliflower (enough)
- spring vegetable salad (2 cups)

Dinner
- Jamaican red pea soup* (2 cups)
- fruit (1 medium pear)

Exercise
Level 1
- Warm up. Start with a five-minute walk at a moderate pace.
- Walk for sixty seconds at a revved-up pace.
- Walk for thirty seconds at a moderate pace.
- Repeat ten times.
- Do calf raises, three sets, twelve to fifteen repetitions.
- Cool down. End with a five-minute walk at an easy pace.

Level 2
- Warm up. Start with a five-minute walk at a moderate pace.
- Walk for sixty seconds at a revved-up pace.
- Walk for thirty seconds at a moderate pace.
- Repeat twelve times.

- Do standing leg curls, three sets, twelve to fifteen repetitions.
- Cool down. End with a five-minute walk at an easy pace.

Level 3

- Warm up. Start with a five-minute walk at a moderate pace.
- Walk for sixty seconds at a revved-up pace.
- Walk for thirty seconds at a moderate pace.
- Repeat fifteen times.
- Do side hip raises, three sets, fifteen to twenty repetitions.
- Cool down. End with a five-minute walk at an easy pace.

Meditation

- Meditate on this quote by Audrey Hepburn: "Nothing is impossible; the word itself says, 'I'm possible!'" Replace the negative thoughts with the serenity prayer: "God grant me the serenity to accept the things I cannot change, courage to change the things I can, and the wisdom to know the difference."

Health Facts—Restorative Sleep

- Restful sleep for at least seven hours per night is essential for good health.
- The body repairs and restores damaged tissues and cells during sleep.
- Information learned during the day is processed and made permanent during sleep. Therefore, sleep deprivation may place you at risk for poor performance and poor memory.
- People who get little sleep are usually slightly more overweight and have shorter life spans than people who get adequate sleep. Sleep and metabolism are controlled by the same area in the brain. Sleep helps maintain a healthy balance of the hormones that make you feel hungry (ghrelin) and full (leptin). When you are sleep-deprived, your level of ghrelin goes up and the level of leptin goes down. This then leads to the desire to overeat, and

the risk of obesity increases. Studies have shown that dieters who were well rested lost more weight.

- Adequate sleep is vital for heart health. Studies have shown that C-reactive protein, which is associated with heart attack risk, was higher in people who got six or fewer hours of sleep at night; this means that lack of adequate amounts of sleep increases your risk of heart attack.

- Adequate sleep reduces stress. During sleep, the production of stress hormones (cortisol and epinephrine) is suppressed. This has a positive effect on blood pressure level, stress, and overall cardiovascular health. In contrast, lack of sleep has an adverse effect on blood pressure and cardiovascular health.

- Research has shown that sleeping in a dark room will increase melatonin production. Melatonin is a hormone that promotes drowsiness and may increase your quality of sleep.

- Watch "Sleep and Restoration" from the *Get Healthy with Dr. Cooper* DVD series.

Document
- Keeping track of your progress is important:
  weight _____ BP_____ BS_____.

Daily Lesson
- Just imagine what would happen to someone who did not sleep for several days. Remember, "Early to bed and early to rise makes a man healthy, wealthy, and wise," according to Benjamin Franklin.

DAY 6

Breakfast
- green smoothie (2 cups)
- walnuts (2 ounces)

Lunch
- roasted vegetables with tofu* (2 cups)
- seasoned edamame (1/4 cup)
- fruits (10 grapes)

Dinner
- hummus* (1/2 cup)
- raw vegetables
- pear (1 medium)

Exercise
Level 1
- Warm up. Start with a seven-minute walk at a moderate pace.
- Run in place, three sets, thirty seconds.
- Do air squats, three sets, twelve to fifteen repetitions.
- Do wall push-ups, three sets, eight to twelve repetitions.
- Do crunches, three sets, twelve to fifteen repetitions.
- Cool down. End with a seven-minute walk at an easy pace.

Level 2
- Warm up. Start with a seven-minute walk at a moderate pace.
- Run in place, three sets, thirty seconds.
- Do air squats, three sets, twelve to fifteen repetitions.
- Do wall push-ups, three sets, eight to twelve repetitions.
- Do crunches, three sets, twelve to fifteen repetitions.
- Cool down. End with a seven-minute walk at an easy pace.

Level 3

- Warm up. Start with a seven-minute walk at a moderate pace.
- Do burpee jacks, three sets, thirty seconds.
- Do kettlebell squats, three sets, twelve to fifteen repetitions.
- Do bridges, three sets, twelve to fifteen repetitions.
- Do planks, three sets, fifteen seconds.
- Cool down. End with a seven-minute walk at an easy pace.

Meditation

- Meditate on how to resist the temptation to overeat and the importance of teaching children good and important values. Read Proverbs 25:16: "Have you found honey? Eat only as much as you need, lest you be filled with it and vomit." And read Proverbs 22:6, "Train up a child in the way he should go, and when he is old he will not depart from it."

Health Facts—A Generation of Obese Children

- The US Department of Health and Human Services reported that one in every three children and adolescents ages six years to nineteen years old is either overweight or obese.
- Obese children are at risk of developing the following diseases: diabetes, high cholesterol, hypertension, arthritis, and even heart disease. If the obesity epidemic continues, then these children will have a shorter life span than that of their parents.
- Poor nutrition and overeating are not the only factors for the obesity crisis; inactivity plays a significant role as well. Only one in three children in the United States is physically active every day. Children now spend at least seven hours daily in front of a screen (TV, computer, video games).
- Parents play a significant role in assisting children in developing good behaviors. Modeling good lifestyle habits is of utmost importance in saving children from chronic diseases. So here are some steps for parents to follow: 1. Plan family activities that will allow the children, as well as the entire family, to become

more physically active, such as swimming, hiking, walking, and biking. 2. Make a conscious effort to reduce the time you and the family spend in sedentary activities, such as watching television and playing video games. 3. Prepare healthy meals ahead of time and spend time to eat together as a family. 4. Expose the family to healthy food choices; provide fruits and vegetables at all meals. 5. Make healthy lifestyle choices and habits for the entire family.

- Modeling healthy lifestyle habits will assist with the transformation of your children into healthy adults.
- Watch "Maintaining a Healthy Weight" from the *Get Healthy with Dr. Cooper* DVD series (www.cooperwellnesscenter.com).

Document

- Log your progress: weight _____ BP_____ BS_____.

Daily Lesson

- Eat to maintain good health. Modeling healthy eating habits as well as healthy lifestyle habits in general is of utmost importance to building a healthier generation!

DAY 7

Breakfast

- blueberry whole wheat pancake* (1)
- fruit sauce (2 tablespoons)
- peanuts (1 ounce)
- cantaloupe (1 cup)

Lunch

- Jamaican stew peas* (1/2 cup)
- brown rice (1/2 cup)
- stir-fry cabbage and carrot (1/2 cup)
- green leafy vegetable salad (2 cups)
- fresh fruit (1 pear)

Dinner

- cream of pumpkin soup* (2 cups)
- raw vegetables (2 cups)

Exercise

Rest today.

Keys to a Good Night's Rest

1. Develop a routine. Strive to go to bed about the same time every night.
2. Turn off the lights. Darkness improves melatonin production, which enhances sleep.
3. Keep the room quiet. Turn off the television and put away all electronics.
4. Keep the room well ventilated and comfortable.
5. No meals or drinks four to five hours prior to bedtime.
6. Avoid coffee. This is a stimulant; it will decrease your ability to fall asleep.

7. Avoid all sleep aids; you will become dependent on these drugs, and your body will lose the ability to fall asleep naturally.

8. Avoid physical exercise just before bedtime. This will increase energy and may delay the onset of sleep.

9. Be in bed about two hours before midnight. The benefits from growth hormone and tissue repair surge at about ten at night.

10. Get a minimum of seven to eight hours of undisturbed sleep each night. Adequate rest improves memory and decreases the risk of obesity, diabetes, and hypertension.

11. Develop a forgiving spirit. Reflect on the positives, and be optimistic. End your day in meditation or prayer.

12. Get up the same time each morning. Start your day feeling rested and energized to face the challenges of a new day.

Meditation

- Spend twenty to thirty minutes today in deep meditation, thinking of things that are positive and uplifting. Read Philippians 4:8: "Finally, brethren, whatever things are true, whatever things *are* noble, whatever things *are* just, whatever things *are* pure, whatever things *are* lovely, whatever things *are* of good report, if *there is* any virtue and if *there is* anything praiseworthy—meditate on these things."

Health Facts—Emotions and Health

- Scientists have discovered that people who are optimistic build a stronger immune system, recover faster from illnesses, and in general, live longer and happier lives than those who are pessimistic.

- Humans are emotional beings who experience a range of emotions from extreme happiness or joy to sadness or depression. Every thought that we think has a physiological effect on our bodies that will promote either health or illness. Brokenness, such as depression, anxiety, stress, unhappiness, anger, hostility, loneliness, pessimism, and lack of love, may lead to poor health.

- Negative emotion may stimulate the production of chemicals, such as catecholamine and cortisol, which then may lead to the production of hypertension, elevated heart rate, elevated blood sugar, and even cardiovascular disease.
- People with negative emotions may also experience generalized joint and muscle pain as a result of increased inflammation in the joints and muscles.
- When the body is in a state of negative emotions, you will not enjoy a sense of well-being; however, when these emotions are converted to positive ones, this will stimulate the brain to produce hormones like serotonin and dopamine. These hormones then will produce a sense of well-being and relaxation. You will feel more at peace, and some of these negative symptoms, such as pain and stiffness, will be relieved.
- Here are some positive emotions that are linked with good health and longevity: encouragement, hope, faith, sympathy, optimism, happiness, forgiveness, and love.
- Watch "The Mind-Body Connection" from the *Get Healthy with Dr. Cooper* DVD series.

Document
- Weight_____ BP_____ BS_____.

Daily Lesson
- Be infectious with positive emotions today and strive to build a relationship with family and friends as well as the Creator.

DAY 8

Breakfast
- old-fashioned oats (1 cup)
- walnuts, nuts (2 ounces)
- fruits (1/4 cup mixed berries)

Lunch
- bean burritos* (2)
- mango avocado salad* (1 cup)

Dinner
- quinoa salad* (2 cups)
- mixed nuts (1 ounce)
- apple (1 medium)

Exercise
Level 1
- Warm up. Start with a five-minute walk at a moderate pace.
- Walk for sixty seconds at a revved-up pace.
- Walk for thirty seconds at a moderate pace.
- Repeat ten times.
- Do hamstring and quad stretches, two sets, fifteen seconds.
- Cool down. End with a five-minute walk at an easy pace.

Level 2
- Warm up. Start with a five-minute walk at a moderate pace.
- Walk for sixty seconds at a revved-up pace.
- Walk for thirty seconds at a moderate pace.
- Repeat ten times.
- Do planks, three sets, fifteen seconds.
- Cool down. End with a five-minute walk at an easy pace.

Level 3

- Warm up. Start with a five-minute walk at a moderate pace.
- Walk for sixty seconds at a revved-up pace.
- Walk for thirty seconds at a moderate pace.
- Repeat ten times.
- Do side-to-side squat jumps, four sets, fifteen to twenty repetitions.
- Cool down. End with a five-minute walk at an easy pace.

Meditation

- Think about someone you need to forgive or something negative that you need to let go of. Spend time with positive people today. Read Ephesians 4:31–32: "Let all bitterness, wrath, anger, clamor, and evil speaking be put away from you, with all malice. And be kind to one another, tenderhearted, forgiving one another, even as God in Christ forgave you."

Health Facts—Anger Kills

- Negative thoughts, such as anger, lack of forgiveness, and hate have detrimental effects on health. These negative emotions may lead to overeating, obesity, hypertension, and cardiovascular disease and death.
- Anger is a normal emotion that triggers the well-known fight-or-flight response, preparing us to defend ourselves psychologically and physically in a conflict. The danger is unresolved anger, which is harmful to your health.
- Anger stimulates an increased production of stress hormones, which, over time, could be harmful to your health. The chronic elevation of these stress hormones may weaken the immune system and lead to many health problems, such as headache, digestive problems, insomnia, increased anxiety, depression, high blood pressure, heart attack, and stroke.
- Anger is also associated with other negative emotions, such as bitterness, hopelessness, and sadness.

- Anger can be a precursor to hate and lack of forgiveness. These negative emotional factors are among the most important contribution factors for all diseases, including cancer.
- The Centers for Disease Control and Prevention (CDC) stated that 85 percent of all diseases appear to have an emotional element.
- Effectively managing emotional stress is of utmost importance in disease prevention and for overall optimal health and longevity. Here are some techniques that you may use to manage stress: 1. *confrontation*, assess the reason for the anger and the need for healing; 2. *relaxation*, implement slow and deep breathing, meditation, prayer, and positive thoughts; 3. *mending*, beginning to forgive and rebuild relationships (seek professional help if necessary); 4. *taking charge*, daily regular physical exercise, yoga, developing a positive attitude; 5. *reinforcement*, surrounding yourself with positive people and continuing to implement these techniques.
- Watch "The Mind-Body Connection" from the *Get Healthy with Dr. Cooper* DVD series.

Document
- List one negative thought that you wish to change: _____
  Weight _____ BP_____ BS_____

Daily Lesson
- Life is too short to live with anger. Refusing to forgive is like a cancer that is slowly destroying your health.

Day 9

Breakfast
- Dr. Cooper's famous breakfast granola (1 cup)
- nondairy milk (1 cup)
- fresh fruits (2 plums)

Lunch
- raw vegetables (abundant)
- eggplant roll-ups (4)
- fresh fruit (1/2 cup papaya)

Dinner
- hummus and vegetable sticks
- oat fruit smoothie*

Exercise

Level 1
- Warm up. Start with a seven-minute walk at a moderate pace.
- Do kettlebell squats, three sets, twelve to fifteen repetitions.
- Do the all-four kick-backs, three sets, twelve to fifteen repetitions.
- Do push-ups, three sets, eight to twelve repetitions.
- Do the bicycle, three sets, thirty seconds.
- Cool down. End with a seven-minute walk at an easy pace.

Level 2
- Warm up. Start with a seven-minute walk at a moderate pace.
- Do squats with twist, three sets, twelve to fifteen repetitions.
- Do reverse lunges with weight, three sets, twelve to fifteen repetitions.
- Do triceps dips, three sets, fifteen to twenty repetitions.
- Do high knees, three sets, thirty seconds.
- Cool down. End with a seven-minute walk at an easy pace.

Level 3

- Warm up. Start with a seven-minute walk at a moderate pace.
- Do burpee jacks, four sets, thirty seconds.
- Do mountain climbers, four sets, thirty seconds.
- Do triceps extensions, four sets, fifteen to twenty repetitions.
- Do side bridges, four sets, thirty to forty-five seconds.
- Cool down. End with a seven-minute walk at an easy pace.

Meditation

- Meditate for twenty to thirty minutes on how to stay focused on the healthy lifestyle that you have chosen. Begin to envision the big picture—less medication or probably no medication and overall improved health. Read Jeremiah 29:11: "For I know the thoughts that I think toward you, says the LORD, thoughts of peace and not of evil, to give you a future and a hope."

Health Facts—Preventive Screening

- In order to maintain good health, prevention of disease is no doubt the best secret and early detection is important.
- Early diagnosis of certain diseases, such as cancer, leads to better and more effective management, which could sometimes mean a complete cure.
- Everyone should visit his or her health care provider at least once a year for a general evaluation and screening. For those of you who are being treated for any medical condition, visits with your health care provider should be more frequent.
- Discuss with your health care provider about what preventive health screening is needed for your age and then follow through on the suggestion. Here are some routine screenings that you should be aware of:
  - Mammograms are used to screen for breast cancer. The screening is usually done yearly in woman ages forty to about eighty-five years, unless otherwise indicated.

- Colon cancer screening—some of the methods used are colonoscopy and flexible sigmoidoscopy or checking stool for occult blood. Screening for colorectal cancer usually starts at age fifty unless there is a family history of colon cancer; then the initial screening is usually done ten years earlier than the age of the youngest person to be diagnosed with colon cancer in that family.
- Pap smear—this test is done to diagnose cancer of the cervix. It is recommended for all women who are sexually active. This test is done yearly or sometimes every two years. It is not recommended for women who have had a hysterectomy or those who are about seventy years old unless otherwise indicated.
- Prostate cancer screening—for men ages forty-five years old and above, a yearly digital rectal exam and obtaining the level for the prostate-specific antigen (PSA) is recommended.

- Vaccines or immunizations you need include the following:
  - The influenza or flu vaccine is usually given during the months of September through April. It is recommended for all persons except those who are allergic to eggs.
  - The hepatitis B vaccine is recommended for all health care providers or anyone whose job entails exposure to blood or blood products.
  - The pneumonia vaccine is recommended for anyone ages sixty-five and above or at any age after splenectomy (removal of the spleen). This vaccine is usually given once in a lifetime.
- Watch "The Prevention of Cancer" from the *Get Healthy with Dr. Cooper* DVD series.

Document

- Weight _____ BP_____ BS_____

Daily Lesson

- This race is not a sprint but a marathon; thus it is not for the swift but for those who will endure to the end. So *press on*!

DAY 10

Breakfast

- bran cereal (1 cup)
- mixed berries (1/2 cup)
- walnuts (2 ounces)
- flaxseed (2 tablespoons)
- almond or soy milk (1 cup)

Lunch

- lentil burger* served with lettuce and tomato
- sweet potato fries* (1 cup)
- apple (1 medium)

Dinner

- raw vegetables (2 cups)
- three-bean chili (1cup)
- fresh fruit (1 kiwi)

Exercise

Level 1

- Warm up. Start with a five-minute walk at a moderate pace.
- Walk for sixty seconds at a revved-up pace.
- Walk for thirty seconds at a moderate pace.
- Repeat ten times.
- Do hamstring and quad stretch, two sets, fifteen seconds.
- Cool down. End with a five-minute walk at an easy pace.

Level 2

- Warm up. Start with a five-minute walk at a moderate pace.
- Walk for sixty seconds at a revved-up pace.
- Walk for thirty seconds at a moderate pace.
- Repeat ten times.

- Do planks, three sets, fifteen seconds.
- Cool down. End with a five-minute walk at an easy pace.

Level 3

- Warm up. Start with a five-minute walk at a moderate pace.
- Walk for sixty seconds at a revved-up pace.
- Walk for thirty seconds at a moderate pace.
- Repeat ten times.
- Do side-to-side squat jumps, four sets, fifteen to twenty repetitions.
- Cool down. End with a five-minute walk at an easy pace.

Meditation

- Think of someone whose life you would like to bless today as you share an act of love or kindness. Read Acts 20:35: "I have shown you in every way, by laboring like this, that you must support the weak. And remember the words of the Lord Jesus, that He said, 'It is more blessed to give than to receive.'"

Health Facts—The Benefits of Good Relationships

- The World Health Organization defines health as a state of complete physical, mental, and social well-being and not merely the absence of disease or infirmity. Therefore, in order to achieve complete health, all three aspects—physical, mental, and social—must be addressed. Studies have shown that people without strong social bonds enjoy poor health, which predisposes them to a much shorter life span.
- Studies show that social relationships have long-term and short-term effects on health that could either promote good health or cause illness. These effects emerge in childhood and cascade down throughout life to foster cumulative advantage and disadvantage in health. Social relationships, both quantity and quality, affect mental health, health behavior, physical health, and mortality risk.

- We are social beings, and therefore, the support of others is a very important aspect of health. Dr. Erik Peper from San Francisco University states, "There is overwhelming evidence that people who have few social contacts are more likely to get ill and less likely to recover from an illness."
- A study done by the University of Michigan in 2013 showed that one of the risk factors for becoming depressed is the *quality* of the relationships people have with one another. One unconventional treatment that has seemed to be effective for depression is spending time with positive people, taking care of animals, or helping someone in need.
- Researchers have also found that providing social support to others may have positive effects on people suffering from heart disease, neurological conditions, and emotional disorders, such as anxiety, depression, stress-related conditions, and even cancer.
- Studies have shown that strong social connectedness is pivotal to good health—mental, psychological, and physical.
- Social isolation shortens your life span by up to ten years.
- Watch "Is Your Lifestyle Killing You?" from the *Get Healthy with Dr. Cooper* DVD series.

Document
- Weight _____ BP _____ BS _____

Daily Lesson
- Focus on your relationships. Begin to form tighter bonds with family and friends.

Day 11

Breakfast
- French toast* (1 slice)
- fruit salad (1 cup)
- cashew nuts (2 ounces)
- flaxseed (2 tablespoons)

Lunch
- vegetable wrap* (1 serving)
- cream of broccoli soup* (1 cup)
- fresh fruit (1 medium peach)

Dinner
- hummus* (1/2 cup)
- carrots, celery, and zucchini (2 cups)
- Dr. Cooper's famous banana peanut butter ice cream* (2 scoops)

Exercise
Level 1
- Warm up. Start with a seven-minute walk at a moderate pace.
- Do kettlebell squats, three sets, twelve to fifteen repetitions.
- Do all-four kick-backs, three sets, twelve to fifteen repetitions.
- Do push-ups, three sets, eight to twelve repetitions.
- Do the bicycle, three sets, thirty seconds.
- Cool down. End with a seven-minute walk at an easy pace.

Level 2
- Warm up. Start with a seven-minute walk at a moderate pace.
- Do squats with a twist, three sets, twelve to fifteen repetitions.
- Do reverse lunges with weight, three sets, twelve to fifteen repetitions.
- Do triceps dips, three sets, twelve to fifteen repetitions.

- Do high knees, three sets, thirty seconds.
- Cool down. End with a seven-minute walk at an easy pace.

Level 3
- Warm up. Start with a seven-minute walk at a moderate pace.
- Do burpee jacks, four sets, thirty seconds.
- Do mountain climbers, four sets, thirty seconds.
- Do triceps extensions, 4 sets, twelve to fifteen repetitions.
- Do side bridges, four sets, thirty to forty-five seconds.
- Cool down. End with a seven-minute walk at an easy pace.

Meditation
- Meditate on a thought that is usually uplifting and inspiring to you. Read Proverbs 20:1: "Wine is a mocker, strong drink is a brawler, and whoever is led astray is not wise."

Health Fact—The Truth about Alcohol
- The consumption of alcohol and its effect on health is usually controversial. Some believe that consuming a small amount of alcohol is good for your health. While this statement could be correct, the question then is "What is a small or moderate amount of alcohol, and how do you know when to stop?" Thus, it may be safer just to avoid alcohol altogether. Here are some of the health risks from alcohol consumption:
  - High blood pressure—alcohol may disrupt how your blood vessels dilate or constrict in response to stress. Over time, this elevated blood pressure may become chronic and can lead to many health problems, such as heart disease, kidney disease, and stroke.
  - Nutritional deficiencies—some vitamin deficiencies, such as folate and vitamin B1, are usually associated with chronic alcohol abuse. These nutritional deficiencies are associated with anemia, poor heart function, and peripheral neuropathy (painful pins-and-needles-like

feelings or numbness in the extremities as well as muscle weakness and erectile dysfunction).

- Infectious disease—heavy drinking suppresses the immune system and increases the risk of various infections from tuberculosis to sexually transmitted diseases.
- Adverse effects on other organs—alcohol consumption can irritate the stomach lining, thus causing gastritis. You will perceive abdominal pain, bloating, and sometimes vomiting and symptoms of gastritis. Inflammation of the pancreas, pancreatitis, is more severe and could be life threatening. Symptoms are usually severe abdominal pain radiating to the back. It could also be accompanied by severe vomiting and sometimes fever.
- Liver cirrhosis—chronic alcohol abuse can cause inflammation of the liver initially and then hardening of the liver, which is known as cirrhosis. Liver cirrhosis leads to many other health problems, such as anemia, bleeding disorders, liver failure, renal failure, and death.
- Psychosocial effects—chronic alcohol consumption may lead to spousal abuse, dysfunctional families, and overall poor social relationships.
- If you have a problem with alcohol use, find someone you trust and seek help now. If your goal is to obtain good health that will last for a lifetime, alcohol consumption is a habit that you should probably seek to let go of.

Document
- Weight _____ BP_____ BS_____

Daily Lesson

- "No illness which can be treated by diet should be treated by any other means," according to Maimonides.
- In order to obtain amazing and abundant health, you will need to address not only possible changes in your diet but other lifestyle habits that could potentially destroy your health.

DAY 12

Breakfast
- whole wheat waffles* (1)
- fruit sauce* (2 tablespoons)
- peanuts (2 ounces)
- almond or soy milk (1 cup)

Lunch
- brown rice black bean salad* (1/2 cup)
- green salad (2 cups)
- fresh fruits (1 cup melon)

Dinner
- cream of pumpkin soup (2 cups)
- grapefruit (half)
- raw vegetable salad with nonoil dressing

Exercise
Level 1
- Warm up. Start with a five-minute walk at a moderate pace.
- Walk for sixty seconds at a revved-up pace.
- Walk for thirty seconds at a moderate pace.
- Repeat ten times.
- Do hamstring and quad stretches, two sets, fifteen seconds.
- Cool down. End with a five-minute walk at an easy pace.

Level 2
- Warm up. Start with a five-minute walk at a moderate pace.
- Walk for sixty seconds at a revved-up pace.
- Walk for thirty seconds at a moderate pace.
- Repeat ten times.

- Do planks, three sets, fifteen seconds.
- Cool down. End with a five-minute walk at an easy pace.

Level 3
- Warm up. Start with a five-minute walk at a moderate pace.
- Walk for sixty seconds at a revved-up pace.
- Walk for thirty seconds at a moderate pace.
- Repeat ten times.
- Side-to-side squat jumps, four sets, fifteen to twenty repetitions.
- Cool down. End with five-minute walk at an easy pace.

Meditation
- Spend twenty to thirty minutes on the power of self-control and why a lifestyle free of alcohol and smoking is important for your success. Read Proverbs 3:1–2: "My son, do not forget my law, but let your heart keep my commandments; for length of days and long life and peace they will add to you."

Health Facts—Tobacco Use
- Over the last several decades, the number of adults who smoke tobacco has significantly decreased from a high of over 40 percent in 1965 to as low as 16.7 percent in 2018 according to the CDC (CDC.gov).
- Tobacco smoking has been found to be harmful to almost every organ in the body and diminishes a person's overall health.
- There are many cancer-causing chemicals in tobacco smoke, some of which are benzene, aromatic amines, chromium, tobacco-specific nitrosamines, polycyclic aromatic hydrocarbons, and arsenic.
- Some of the common diseases that are associated with smoking are chronic obstructive pulmonary disease (COPD), emphysema, chronic bronchitis, osteoporosis, worsening of asthma symptoms in adults, and peripheral vascular disease.

- Smoking is the leading cause of cancer and cancer-related deaths. Smoking causes cancers, such as lung, esophagus, larynx, mouth, throat, kidney, bladder, and stomach, just to name a few.
- Smoking makes it harder for women to get pregnant. Women who smoke during pregnancy have a higher risk of miscarriage or having an ectopic pregnancy or premature delivery.
- Secondhand smokers—otherwise known as passive smokers— are at risk for some of the same diseases seen in active smokers. Secondhand smokers have increased risk for lung cancer, cardiovascular disease, and complications during pregnancy and death.
- There is hope after quitting smoking. Quitting smoking lowers cancer risk. Studies have shown that people who quit smoking, regardless of age, are less likely to die from smoking-related illnesses than those who continue to smoke.
- For information on how to quit smoking, you may visit the website smokefree.gov.
- As you seek to embrace a healthier lifestyle, there are other substances that you should probably consider eliminating from your lifestyle, such as coffee or caffeinated drinks. Caffeine is a stimulant, which could increase your blood pressure and your heart rate.

Document
- Weight _____ BP _____ BS _____
- Write one habit you wish to get rid of _____

Daily Lesson
- In order to obtain amazing and abundant health, you will need to address not only possible changes in your diet but other lifestyle habits that could potentially destroy your health.

Day 13

Breakfast
- old-fashioned oats (1 cup)
- chopped strawberries (1/4 cup)
- walnuts (1 ounce)

Lunch
- tofu eggless sandwich* (1)
- raw vegetables (2 cups)
- apple (1 medium)

Dinner
- cold summer soup* (2 cups)
- bean dip (1/2 cup)
- whole wheat pita chips (1 serving)

Exercise

Level 1
- Warm up. Start with a seven-minute walk at a moderate pace.
- Do kettlebell squats, three sets, fifteen to twenty repetitions.
- Do all-four kick-backs, three sets, fifteen to twenty repetitions.
- Do push-ups, three sets, eight to twelve repetitions.
- Do the bicycle, three sets, thirty seconds.
- Cool down. End with a seven-minute walk at an easy pace.

Level 2
- Warm up. Start with a seven-minute walk at a moderate pace.
- Do squats with a twist, three sets, fifteen to twenty repetitions.
- Do reverse lunges with weights, three sets, fifteen to twenty repetitions.
- Do triceps dips, three sets, fifteen to twenty repetitions.

- Do high knees, three sets, thirty seconds.
- Cool down. End with a seven-minute walk at an easy pace.

Level 3

- Warm up. Start with a seven-minute walk at a moderate pace.
- Do burpee jacks, four sets, thirty seconds.
- Do mountain climbers, four sets, thirty seconds.
- Do triceps extensions, four sets, fifteen to twenty repetitions.
- Do side bridges, four sets, thirty to forty-five seconds.
- Cool down. End with a seven-minute walk at an easy pace.

Meditation

- Spend twenty to thirty minutes in meditation on where you see yourself in the future as you adopt this new lifestyle makeover. Trust in yourself and in the higher power that success will be yours. Read Philippians 4:13: "I can do all things through Christ who strengthens me."

Health Fact—Faith and Health

- Though difficult to quantify, researchers are still trying to explain the link between faith and healing. Thus far, they have seen a positive link to reduction in blood pressure and heart disease risk in patients who practice prayer and meditation. These patients also have a stronger immune system, and there is a reduction of anxiety and depression.
- Faith is a belief or trust in the divine power (God), while spirituality is an attachment to religious value. Studies like the Alameda County study have shown that frequent attendance at religious services decreases mortality. People who belong to a faith community tend to have improved health practices; they also have more social contacts and more stable marriages. All these factors have a positive effect on promoting good health.
- Many studies have explored the effect of religion and faith on mental health, such as depression and anxiety. The conclusion

showed a small effect but an association between the two; the more religious a person was, the fewer symptoms of depression he or she experienced.

- Researchers have also looked at the relationship between religion or spirituality and adolescent substance abuse, anxiety, depression, delinquency, and suicidal behavior. The researchers were able to determine that there is a significant relationship between religiousness and improved mental health.

- Furthermore, regular church attendees or people of faith usually have a sense of purpose; they have hope in a higher power, and these church attendees feel loved and supported, knowing that they are never alone. These factors promote positive emotions essential for good health.

- People who pray or meditate regularly tend to live longer and healthier lives.

Document

- Weight _____ BP_____ BS_____
- Health goals: _____

Daily Lesson

- Make practicing good health a habit. Educate yourself, meditate daily, join a faith community, and develop a routine that will make this a success.

DAY 14

Breakfast
- scrambled tofu with kale* (1/2)
- baked sweet potato (1 medium)
- grapefruit (half)

Lunch
- Thai curry tofu* (1/2 cup)
- brown rice (1/2 cup)
- mixed vegetable salad with walnuts* (2 cups)

Dinner
- lentil soup* (2 cups)
- fresh fruit bowl (cut apple, cantaloupe, and papaya)

Exercise
Rest today.

Keys to Emotional and Mental Rest
1. Develop a routine and set aside time each day to disconnect from your daily routine and unwind.
2. Put away the electronics; read an uplifting book or get a hobby.
3. Spend some time outdoors and enjoy nature with your family and loved ones.
4. Reach out to a friend; spend some time laughing and reflecting on positive memories.
5. Find a quiet place to relax, close your eyes, and meditate on all the blessings of the day.
6. Maintain a spirit of peace and joy. Express love to those around you.
7. Embrace the healing power of forgiveness and move away from anger.
8. Exercise faith, hope, and trust in a higher power.

Meditation
- Think of ways to share this amazing health journey that you have embarked on with family, friends, and your community at large.

Health Facts—The Blue Zone Phenomenon
- Research shows that there are about five regions in the world in which people are living to one hundred years. These regions are the following:
  - ➢ the Italian island of Sardinia
  - ➢ Okinawa, Japan
  - ➢ Loma Linda, California
  - ➢ Costa Rica's isolated Nicoya Peninsula
  - ➢ Ikaria, an isolated Greek island.
- The people who live in these blue zones no doubt have a secret to a longer and happier life, but don't lose hope! You have just found those precious secrets in this book!
- Let's review some of the good-health practices that will promote longer life:
  - Practice balance in your daily life; enjoy, in moderation, what is good and abstain from what is bad for your health.
  - Let food be your medicine and your medicine be food; select healthy foods and consume enough.
  - Remember exercise is medicine, so become engaged in physical exercise daily.
  - Practice moderation in technology; spend time with family outdoors and enjoy nature.
  - Use your mind carefully and wisely; be positive, be enthusiastic about life, and have a brighter outlook on life.
  - Spend time around positive people and build strong relationships.
  - Develop wholesome behaviors, such as not smoking and avoiding coffee and alcohol.
  - Get spiritually connected.

- Hippocrates wrote, "If someone wishes for good health, one must first ask himself if he is ready to do away with the reasons for his illness. Only then is it possible to help him." In this book, you have the tools that you may use to change your health destiny. However, like Hippocrates states, if you wish to embrace good health, you must first be ready to let go of those habits that would impede you from attaining your full health potential.
- Watch "Healthy Lifestyle" from the *Get Healthy with Dr. Cooper* DVD series (visit www.cooperwellnesscenter.com).

Document

- Weight _____ BP _____ BS_____
  Cholesterol_____ HbA1c_____

Daily Lesson

- This is only the beginning of your journey. Surround yourself with everything that is positive to propel you on your way to success. As you continue this journey, you should use the information you have learned to educate, inspire, and empower others to enjoy the amazing health that you have discovered.

CHAPTER 13

The Makeover Results

*C*ongratulations! You have successfully completed fourteen days of your new and amazing lifestyle makeover. You must be feeling awesome! This is only the beginning of your journey toward longevity and living free from disease. Many have walked this journey before you and have written different stories. Permit me to share one such story with you.

Fifty-nine-year-old Mary Adams came to my office suffering physically and emotionally. Recently diagnosed with breast cancer and thyroid cancer, Mary was undergoing vigorous tests to identify how extensively these cancers were progressing. The reality of her diagnoses was frightening and mentally draining. During this difficult time, she also had diabetes, which was being treated with metformin (Glucophage). Mary was miserable with this drug; she had daily diarrhea and abdominal discomfort. At this point, Mary just wanted to feel physically well so that she could fight the cancers, physically and emotionally.

That day, during the course of her visit with me, I felt her pain, her fear, and her anxiety. As her physician, I wanted her to enjoy health so I gave her the prescription for *Fourteen Days to Amazing Health*. Initially, she was hesitant. She thought that changing her lifestyle would be difficult, but she reluctantly agreed to proceed with the plan. I took her off the metformin and started her on the plant-based diet plan.

She returned to my office fourteen days later in great amazement. Her diarrhea and abdominal discomfort were gone, and her blood sugar was within the normal range. She was happier, energized, and ready to face the challenges of the dreaded "C" word, *cancer*. Mary continued to embrace this new lifestyle during chemotherapy and after surgery. In a follow-up visit several weeks later, Mary told me that her oncologist expressed amazement at her improved physical status as well as her emotional and mental readiness to fight the difficulties that might await her as she continues to deal with the reality of the two cancers.

The *Fourteen Days to Amazing Health* program is only a jump-start to the new and better you. It is the beginning of your journey on your quest to a longer, happier, and healthier life. The positive changes that you experience with your health, whether that be weight loss, improved blood sugar levels, improved cholesterol levels, or a decrease in the number of medications you take, should motivate and inspire you to continuing this journey for more than fourteen days.

Table Showing Weight Reduction After Twelve Weeks

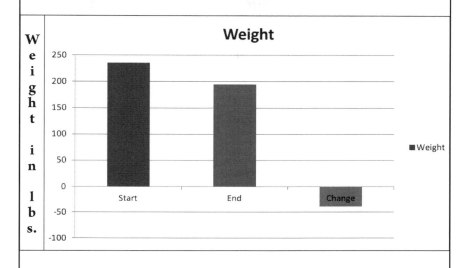

This graph reflects the average weight reduction seen in 137 patients who were enrolled in my twelve-week wellness program at Cooper Wellness Center.

This graph represents improvement in Total Cholesterol after twelve weeks.

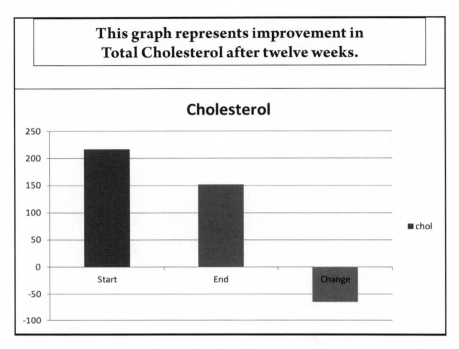

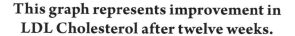

**This graph represents improvement in
LDL Cholesterol after twelve weeks.**

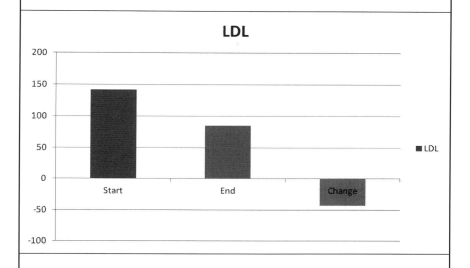

These graphs reflect the average total cholesterol and LDL cholesterol reduction for 127 patients enrolled in my twelve-week wellness program. Many of these patients continue to do well with reduced medication and some are even off all cholesterol medications.

This graph represents improvement in Blood Pressure after twelve weeks.

BLOOD PRESSURE

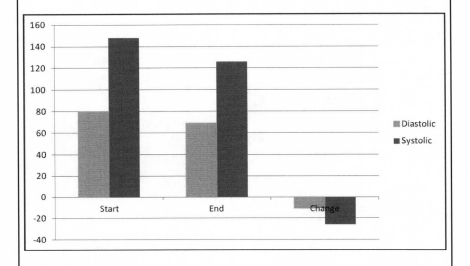

This graph represents the average blood pressure drop in 116 patients enrolled at Cooper Wellness Center's twelve-week program from 2013 to 2015. Some patients remain off medications while others have reduced their blood pressure medications.

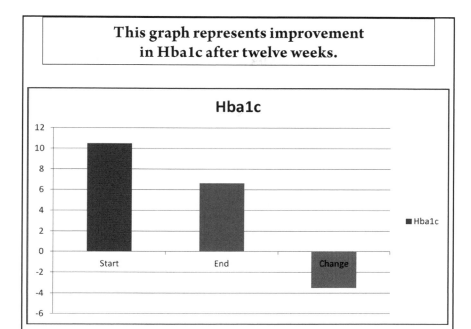

This graph represents improvement in Hba1c after twelve weeks.

This graph represents an average of the change seen in the diabetic patients enrolled in my twelve-week wellness program. Some patients are doing well off all medications, while others have had their medications reduced.

STAYING ON TRACK TO MAINTAIN YOUR GOAL FOR LIFE

Many have walked this road before you. I have patients who, years after changing their lifestyle, have remained off diabetes and cholesterol medication and continue to maintain a healthy weight. However, maintaining the change is not always easy, so here are a few helpful suggestions.

STOCK UP WITH HEALTHY FOODS

There will be times when you will have the desire to eat something that may not be healthy. But if you only have healthy food choices at home, then that will automatically solve the problem. Having healthy food choices on hand will lessen the temptation to reach for any unhealthy option. It is a great idea to keep nuts, seeds, and fresh and dried fruits at home and at work.

CHOOSE WISELY WHEN EATING OUT

It is becoming easier to find healthy meals at restaurants. Many restaurants are now adding vegan or vegetarian options to their menus. Do not hesitate to ask for these options if you do not readily spot them on the menu. Most restaurants will accommodate you. Here are some tips when eating out.

Salads

Be careful with the dressing. You should avoid the use of ranch dressing, as ranch dressing is high in fat. If you decide to have salad dressing, then use a light Italian or vinaigrette dressing and remember to limit the amount that you pour on the salad. Avoid the toppings of bacon, cheese, and croutons. These are high in calories and saturated fat, and you do not want to convert a healthy salad into a meal that will increase your risk of chronic disease. So top your salad with a generous amount of beans, peas, nuts, and seeds, then you will have a complete meal that is filled with vitamins, minerals, phytochemicals, proteins, and good fats and carbohydrates. This type of salad will not only satisfy your hunger but protect you from overeating and fill you for a longer period.

Italian Cuisine

Italian menus are usually great options; however, you must take care, as many of the dishes are prepared with cheese and large amounts of oil. In order to make your dish healthier, ask for whole wheat pasta, if possible. Use vegetables in the pasta. Use marinara sauce instead of Alfredo sauce, and add to your order a bowl of minestrone soup with vegetable broth.

Mexican Cuisine

If you are dining at a Mexican restaurant, be sure to ask if the meals are prepared with lard; this is pork fat, a form of saturated fat that is not good for your overall health. Once you have clarified this, here are some great options: bean burritos, rice and beans with chopped lettuce and tomato on the side, and bean enchiladas. Be careful with the sauce, usually enchiladas are topped with cheese sauce. Tamales made from vegetables or beans and tacos made with potatoes or beans are also good options.

Asian Cuisine

It is very easy to find healthy vegan choices in an Asian restaurant. However, the danger is the amount of oil and possibly sugar used in these menus. Some helpful tips are to choose menus with tofu and vegetables, be cautious with the heavy sweet sauces, and fill up your plate with immature legumes, such as snow peas and string beans. Add broccoli and cauliflower to your plate as well.

Indian Cuisine

I enjoy dining at Indian restaurants. Be sure to ask for vegan options, as many of these dishes are made with dairy products, such as yogurt or cream. Some great options are chickpea curry, eggplant curry, lentil soup, and vegetable rice.

AVOID EATING LATE

It appears that eating after five in the evening is a cultural issue, particularly in America, where people are accustomed to having a large meal during the late evening. This is not a healthy habit to perpetuate and is a difficult habit to break. Eating late at night may lead to a poor quality of sleep, obesity, poor blood sugar control, indigestion, esophageal reflux, and chronic cough. If you are struggling with late-evening meals, here are a few tips to minimize some of these problems. First, eat your last meal at or before five. If you have to eat after five, then make that last meal a salad of fruits or vegetables, a bowl of soup, or nondairy yogurt. It would not hurt to go for a short walk after that meal; this will assist in digestion of your meal before bedtime. I also advise my patients not to eat late at night because this will increase the risk of weight gain. During sleep, the body has no time to use the extra calories, and therefore, those calories are stored as adipose tissue (fat tissue), which then leads to weight gain or obesity.

PART 3

Amazing Fitness Program

CHAPTER 14

The Twenty-One-Day Fitness Challenge

*A*s you have seen in the chapter on exercise, active living is paramount to obtaining and maintaining optimal and amazing health. During my wellness program, the participants are encouraged to commit to daily physical exercise for at least six days weekly. Therefore, in order for you to receive the maximum benefit from the program outlined in this book, I have developed a twenty-one-day fitness challenge for you to follow.

There is absolutely no reason to stay physically inactive! Moving your body toward optimal health is quite easy. I have always told my patients that everyone and anyone can participate in some form of physical exercise; the trick to success is the mind. You must first be mentally ready to effect the change that you desire to see in your life. Determination is the key, so even if you are in a wheelchair, bedbound, too overweight to move your legs, or too busy to go to the gym, there is something in this section to engage you.

In this section, there are six days of structured exercise routines, comprising three days of intermittent walking with stretching and three days of full-body workout routines. For maximum benefit, you should complete at least thirty minutes of exercise daily. In order to help you select the correct exercise routine for your level of physical fitness and to prevent injury, the program is structured in three levels. After reviewing the levels, if you are still not certain at what level you should engage, speak with your primary health care provider.

FITNESS LEVELS

Review the levels carefully and then select the one that you are most comfortable with, depending on your current level of fitness.

Level 1

This level is intended for beginners or for those who have never been engaged in physical activity in the past. If you have medical conditions, such as arthritis or lung or heart disease, and have been very hesitant to exercise, then this level is for you. The exercise routines are simple and not very strenuous. Please continue at this level until you feel comfortable to transition to level 2.

Level 2

This level is more physically challenging and is recommended for those who have been engaged in physical exercise in a regular or intermittent manner or for those who have successfully completed level 1. These exercise routines are more intense and demanding on the body.

Level 3

This level is intended for those who are already physically fit but are too busy to go to the gym. The exercise routines in this level are intense and challenging; they will propel you to advance physically. These exercise routines are great to help you keep in shape as you prevent, improve, or reverse chronic diseases.

MAKE FITNESS A HABIT FOR LIFE

The goal of this book is to give you the tools you need to obtain optimal health. Keeping your body physically active is very important. Therefore, staying physically active is a prescription for life. This means that the physical fitness challenge does not end after twenty-one days. Certainly, if you start at level 1 and then move up to level 2, you can stay at this level as long as you desire. Then continue to progress to the subsequent level and find a balance. There may be danger in physical activity, so be careful. Continue to cultivate habits that will propel you on your journey to a long, happy, and more fulfilled life.

Level 1 Full-Body Workout Exercises

running in place

air squats

wall push-ups

crunches

side-to-side squat jump

in-place forward lunges

bicep curls

single leg lifts

burpee jacks

kettlebell squats

bridges

planks

bilateral leg raises / double leg lifts

goblet squat

step-up and kick-back

LEVEL 2 FULL-BODY EXERCISES

kettlebell squats

all four kick-back

push-ups

bicycle

squats

reverse lunge with weight

triceps dips

high knees

burpee jacks

mountain climbers

triceps extensions

side bridges

jumping lunges

squat with kick-backs

the hundred

elevated bridges

squats with a twist

LEVEL 3 FULL-BODY WORKOUT EXERCISES

compound squats

kettlebell lunge with twist

push-ups

triceps dips

kettlebell squats

calf raises

bicep curls

bilateral raises

squat and overhead press

burpee jacks

elevated bridges

planks

kick-back with weights

the criss-cross

corkscrew

Bulgarian split squat

CHAPTER 15

Exercise Routines in Motion

LUNGES

1.   2.   3.

Step 1. Start by standing upright with your feet shoulder-width apart.

Step 2. Step forward with your left foot while keeping your upper body straight throughout the exercise.

Step 3. Lower your body until your left knee is bent about ninety degrees. Your knee should not touch the floor. Push with the left foot to a standing position again. Repeat, stepping forward with the right foot.

Do fifteen to twenty repetitions.

The *lunge* exercise strengthens and tones the muscles of the core and lower extremities and increases the flexibility of the knees. Be cautious if you have any knee problems.

JUMPING LUNGES

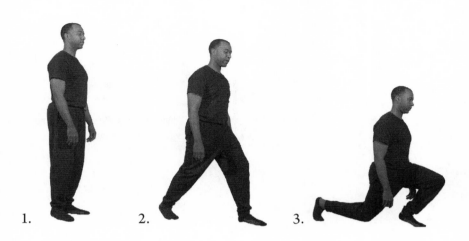

1.   2.   3.

Step 1. Stand upright with feet shoulder-width apart.

Step 2. Step forward with one leg into a wide stance (about one leg distance between feet).

Step 3. Lower your hips until both knees are bent. Make sure not to touch the floor. Then spring or jump up as you switch to the other leg.

Do fifteen to twenty repetitions.

The *jumping lunge* exercise is a more challenging exercise for toning your leg muscles. Avoid this exercise if you have knee dysfunctions.

AIR SQUATS

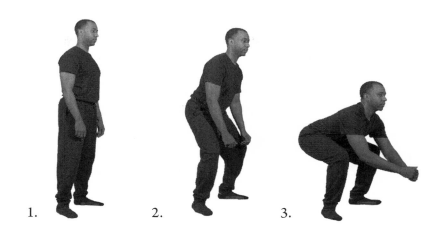

1.   2.   3.

Step 1. Stand upright with feet shoulder-width apart.

Step 2. Slowly bend at the knees as if you were sitting on a chair. Make sure as you are squatting down your heels stay planted on the floor.

Step 3. Squat down slowly until your thighs are parallel to the floor while reaching forward with your arms. Squeeze your buttock muscles and straighten your legs to a standing position.

Do fifteen to twenty repetitions.

Squats, though thought to work the lower body, are in fact a full-body workout. They strengthen the muscles of the lower and upper body, the gluteal muscles, and the core. There are different variations of the squat routine. Be cautious if you have knee dysfunctions.

SQUAT WITH KICK-BACKS

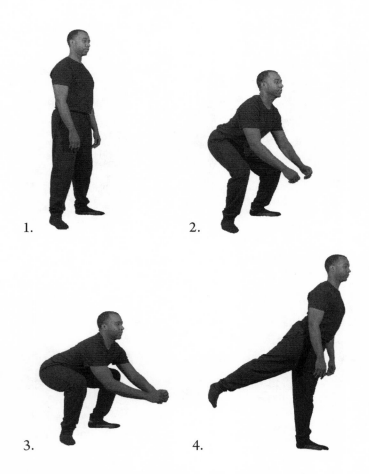

Step 1. Stand upright with feet shoulder-width apart.

Step 2. Slowly bend at the knees as if you were sitting on a chair. Make sure as you are squatting down your heels stay planted on the floor.

Step 3. Squat down until your thighs are parallel to the floor while reaching forward with your arms.

Step 4. Squeeze your buttock muscles and straighten your legs. Raise your torso to stand back up. Resume a standing position. Repeat the squat, shifting your weight to the right side and kicking your left leg backward.

Do fifteen to twenty repetitions.

Here more emphasis is placed on strengthening and building the muscles of the lower body—quadriceps, hamstrings, and gluteal muscles, as well as increasing the flexibility of the knees and hips. However, the muscles of the upper extremities and core are also engaged.

Squat and Press

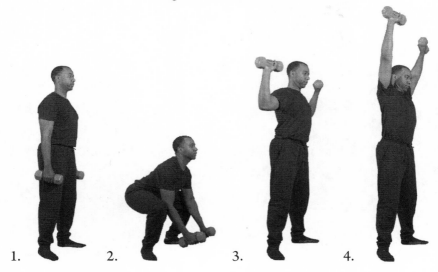

1. 2. 3. 4.

Step 1. Stand upright with feet shoulder-width apart and with weights grasped firmly in each hand.

Step 2. Slowly bend at your knees and squat down. Tighten your abdominal muscles and take deep breaths.

Step 3. After squatting, keep your heels planted on the floor; then return to an upright position, and raise arms with the weights, keeping the shoulders and elbows at a ninety-degree angle.

Step 4. Press up with the weights above your head, keeping the elbows straight. And repeat.

Do fifteen to twenty repetitions.

This is another variation of the squat routine; it is a full-body workout that strengthens and shapes the muscles of the lower and upper body as well as the core.

Caution—Use comfortable weights (three to five pounds) to avoid injury.

ALL-FOUR KICK-BACKS

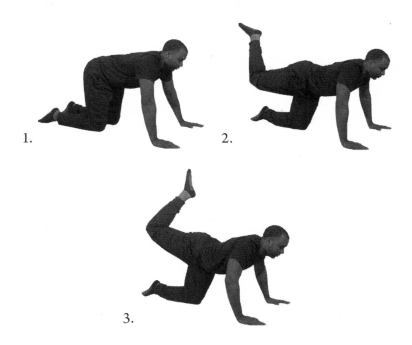

1.

2.

3.

Step 1. Position yourself on your hands, which should be shoulder-width apart, and knees with your back parallel to the floor.

Step 2. Tighten your abdominal muscles, lock your elbows for support, and raise one leg back, keeping the upper leg parallel to the floor and lower leg perpendicular.

Step 3. Keep your gluteal muscles tight. Kick the leg back almost as if you were trying to touch your head with your foot. Then repeat steps 1 and 2 with the other leg.

Do fifteen to twenty repetitions.

The *all-four kick-backs* strengthen and shape the following muscles: lower back, gluteal, quadriceps, and hamstrings. The flexibility of the hips is also improved during this routine.

Knee Highs

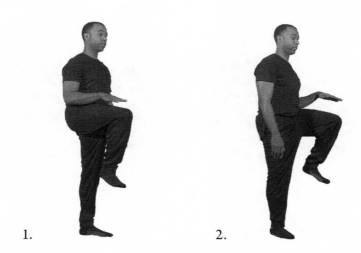

1.   2.

Step 1. Stand with your feet shoulder-width apart, hand at waist level.

Step 2. Shift your weight to the left leg, bring the right knee up to about waist level, and touch your thigh with your right hand.

Step 3. Alternate and do the same thing with the other leg. Make sure you do this at a comfortable pace and keep your abdominal muscles tightened.

This routine can be performed as you run in place. The muscles of the lower body and the abdominals are being strengthened and shaped in the *knee high* exercise, while there is increased flexibility in the hips and knee joints.

Bilateral Leg Raise

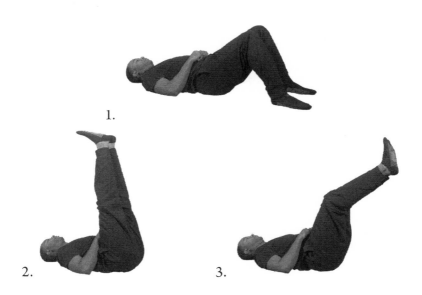

1.

2.

3.

Step 1. Lie straight on your back with your head and back touching the surface and knees slightly bent.

Step 2. Engage your stomach muscles (tighten abs), and raise both legs at the same time, keeping the knees straight and hips at a ninety-degree angle. Hold for one to three seconds at the top.

Step 3. Slowly lower your legs midway before raising them up again. Try to keep your back flat on the floor.

Do twelve to fifteen repetitions, and repeat three times.

This routine strengthens and shapes the muscles of the lower back, the lower body, and the abdominals (abs) while increasing the flexibility and stability of the hips.

Caution—Do not perform the *bilateral leg raise* if you have back problems, unless you have been cleared by your medical practitioner.

PUSH-UP

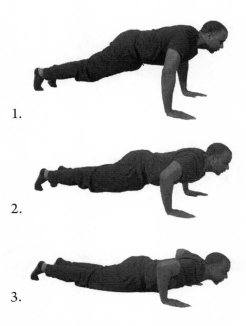

1.

2.

3.

Step 1. Position yourself facedown, supporting your weight on your toes and hands with your palms flat and even with your shoulder level.

Step 2. Tighten your abdominals as you lower your body toward the floor by bending your elbows. Push up with your arms to starting position. Pause in the contracted position. Keep your back straight throughout the exercise.

Step 3. Bring your chest down to the floor, but don't touch the floor. Return to step 2.

The *push-up* exercise works the muscles of the arms, chest, and core.

SIDE BRIDGES

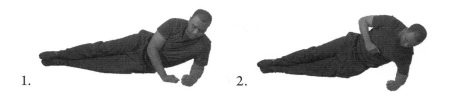

1. 2.

Step 1. While lying on your side with your knees straight and feet together, rest your forearm on the floor.

Step 2. Bring your waist up, and prop your upper body on your elbow and forearm. Brace your core by contracting the abdominal muscles forcefully. Hold your body in a straight line from your head to feet with your elbow directly beneath your shoulder. Hold this position for thirty to forty-five seconds. Return to resting position.

Do five repetitions on each side.

The *side bridge* is an isometric exercise emphasizing the oblique abdominal muscles, the shoulder girdle, and the muscles of the lower back.

Triceps Dips

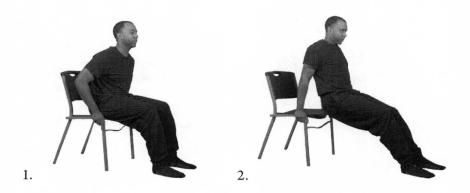

1.   2.

Step 1. On a sturdy chair, place both hands down, grasping on to the edge of the chair.

Step 2. Bend both elbows, lowering your hips as you carry your weight.

Step 3. Press back up, straightening your arms.

Do fifteen to twenty repetitions.

This routine strengthens the muscles of the upper body with special emphasis on the biceps.

BURPEE JACK

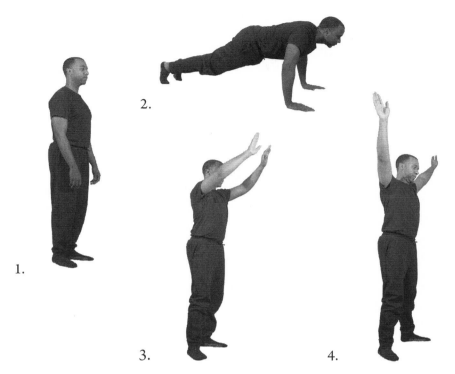

Step 1. Start in an upright position.

Step 2. Go down into a push-up position, and kick your legs back, keeping your back straight.

Step 3. Jump back up to a standing position.

Step 4. Do a jumping jack.

Repeat for thirty seconds and then have a thirty-second break. Do this for two to three minutes.

The *burpee jack* exercise is a full-body workout routine that strengthens and shapes the muscles of the upper and lower body as well as the core and gluteal muscles.

MOUNTAIN CLIMBERS

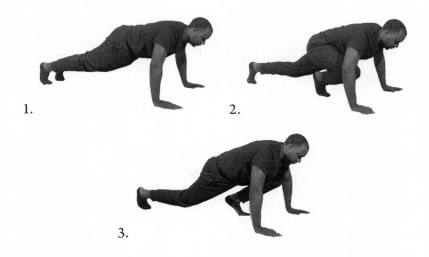

1.

2.

3.

Step 1. Go down to a push-up position with your weight supported by your toes and hands.

Step 2. Bend one knee, and bring it to your chest. Tighten your abdominal muscles, and then straighten the knee and return to your initial position.

Step 3. Now Now repeat the same movement with the other leg (climbing motion).

Do ten repetitions on each side, alternating.

Mountain climbers provide core strengthening and arm and leg strengthening, as well as a cardiovascular workout.

BICYCLES

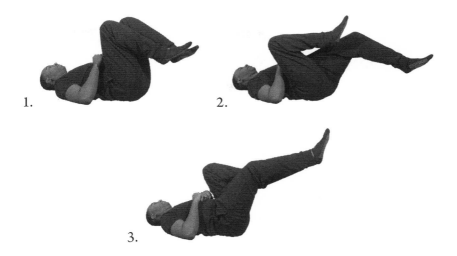

Step 1. Lie on your back with one knee bent up and the other leg straight.

Step 2. Bring one knee toward your chest. Alternate legs up and down, as if you are riding a *bicycle*. Try to keep your back flat on the floor.

Step 3. Keeping your back flat on the floor, point your toes down to enhance muscle strengthening.

Do fifteen to twenty repetitions.

The *bicycle* exercise routine strengthens and tones muscles, such as the quadriceps, hamstrings, and abdominals.

WALL PUSH-UP

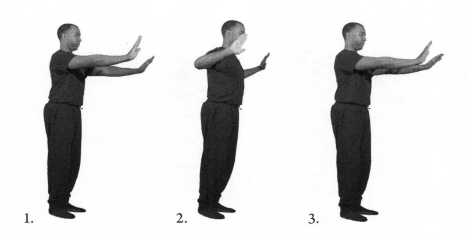

1.   2.   3.

Step 1. Stand facing a wall with your feet about one to two feet back from the wall.

Step 2. Place your hands, palms flat, on the wall, outside shoulder-width apart.

Step 3. Keeping your back straight and your abdominal muscles tight, bend your elbows as you lean forward to touch your nose toward the wall. Push away from the wall by extending your elbows as you return to starting position.

Do fifteen to twenty repetitions and repeat three sets.

This routine is excellent for beginners or for those who want to strengthen chest muscles but have lower back problems.

OVERHEAD TRICEPS EXTENSIONS

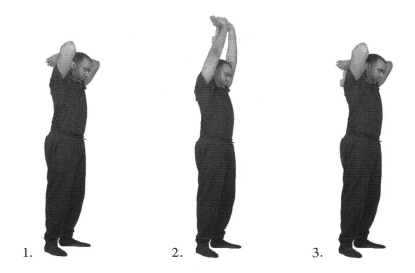

1. 2. 3.

Step 1. Stand with an upright posture, feet shoulder-width apart for a good base of support, while doing these *triceps extension* exercises. Using a dumbbell, place both hands facing up around the top of the dumbbell.

Step 2. Place the dumbbell behind your head and simply extend both arms up toward the ceiling.

Step 3. Then slowly go down behind your head almost until you hit the top of your back and raise your arms up again. Inhale as you bend your elbows, and exhale as you extend them.

Do fifteen to twenty repetitions, and repeat three sets.

The *triceps extension* exercise strengthens and tones the triceps while increasing flexibility of the shoulder and elbow joints.

Bicep Curl

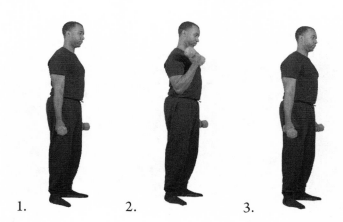

1.　　2.　　3.

Step 1. Stand or sit with good posture to prevent substitution of trunk muscles; keep looking forward while your *biceps* are doing the workout.

Step 2. Grip the dumbbell with your palm facing upward and smoothly curl one elbow at a time, reaching to touch your shoulder. Keep your upper arm pinned to your side.

Step 3. Slowly lower the dumbbell as you extend your arm. Repeat on opposite arm.

Do fifteen to twenty repetitions, three sets.

Select a lightweight dumbbell if you are just starting this exercise; the amount of resistance can easily be increased as your skills progress. Low-resistance weights and a high number of repetitions will build endurance. Higher amounts of weight and a lower number of repetitions build muscle bulk.

HAMSTRING STRETCH

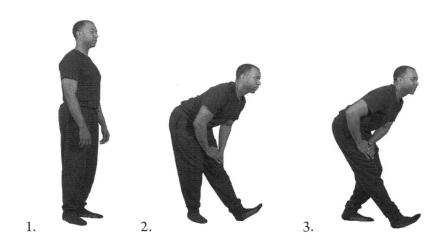

1.   2.   3.

Step 1. Stand upright, and step forward with your right foot, keeping your right heel on the floor, forefoot pointing up.

Step 2. Tighten your abdominals, and bend your left knee slightly to support the weight of your body. Rest your hands on your left thigh for support.

Step 3. Lean forward slightly until you feel a gentle stretch behind your right knee or in your buttocks; hold for fifteen seconds. Alternate steps to stretch the opposite leg. Hold ten seconds while stretching.

Do ten repetitions.

Stretching your *hamstring* muscles can relieve low-back, hip, or knee pain.

Quad Stretch

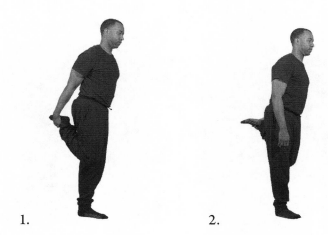

1.   2.

Step 1. Stand with your feet shoulder-width apart. Hold on to a counter or wall for support to avoid losing your balance. Bend your right knee; grasp the ankle with your right hand, and gently pull the foot toward the buttock. Hold as a sustained, steady stretch without bouncing for the count of fifteen to thirty seconds. Repeat to stretch the left quads as well. Hold for ten seconds each.

Do ten repetitions on each leg.

The *quad stretch* exercise strengthens the quadriceps and increases flexibility of the knees.

Glute Stretch

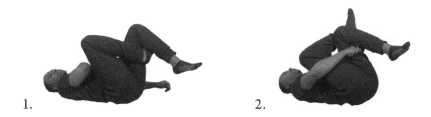

1.   2.

Step 1. Lie on your back with your knees bent.

Step 2. Bend both knees, and bring the right leg in front of the left knee.

Step 3. Grab your left knee with both hands and bring it toward your chest. Use your hands under your left thigh to gently pull your leg toward your chest. (Do not pull against your shin, as this may stress your knee joint.) Gently stretch your buttock by holding steady for fifteen to thirty seconds. Alternate legs to stretch the other gluteal muscles.

Do fifteen to twenty repetitions on each side.

The *glute stretch* exercise works the lower body with special emphasis on the gluteal muscles.

CALF RAISE

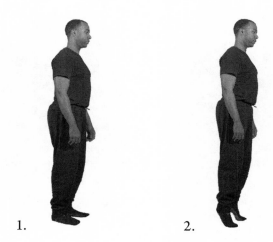

1. 2.

Step 1. Stand with your feet shoulder-width apart. Engage your core by tightening your stomach muscles.

Step 2. Lift your heels off the floor. Stand on your toes for two seconds, and then lower your heels to return to starting position. Remember to inhale as you lift your body and exhale as you lower your body.

Do fifteen to twenty repetitions, three sets.

The *calf raise* exercise strengthens the calf muscles and is very easy to perform.

KETTLEBELL SQUATS/ GOBLET SQUATS

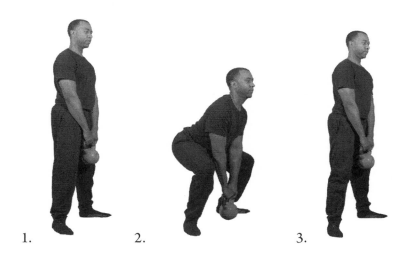

1.   2.   3.

Step 1. Stand upright, feet apart, and hold the kettlebell in front of your legs with two hands. Keep the elbows close to the body. Keep your head and chest up and back straight.

Step 2. Slowly squat down. Keep your heels firmly planted on the floor. Push your hips back until your thighs are parallel to the floor or just below.

Step 3. Return to the standing position and repeat. Inhale as you relax your core, and exhale as you tighten.

Do fifteen to twenty repetitions, three sets.

The *kettlebell / goblet squat* strengthens and tones the muscles of the calf, the hamstrings, gluteals, the obliques, and the biceps. There is also increased flexibility of the hips and knees.

Compound Squat

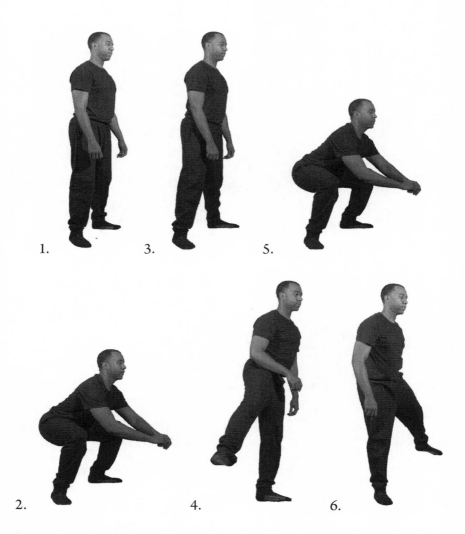

1. 3. 5.

2. 4. 6.

Step 1. Stand upright with your feet shoulder-width apart. Engage your core by pulling in your abdomen.

Step 2. Slowly squat down. Keep your heels firmly planted on the floor. Push your hips back until your thighs are parallel to the floor or just below.

Step 3. Return to a standing position.

Steps 4-5. Move to the right and squat down.

Step 6. Then lift your body up and move to your left and squat down again.

Do fifteen to twenty repetitions, three sets.

The *compound squat* exercise is a full-body workout routine that targets the hamstrings, lower back, calf muscles, abdominals, and gluteals. There is also increased flexibility of the hips and knees.

PLANK

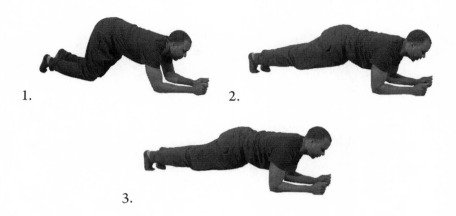

1.

2.

3.

Step 1. With your forearms on the floor, get into a push-up position. Keep your weight on the elbows and forearms. The body should form a straight line from the shoulders to the ankles.

Steps 2-3. Hold yourself up for fifteen to twenty seconds and increase your hold time as you get better. Keep your abdominal muscles (core) tightened.

Repeat three times.

The *plank* exercise helps to strengthen and shape the muscles of your core as well as the upper and lower body. Some of the target muscles are the deltoids, biceps, triceps, abdominals, pectorals, the gluteus maximus, quadriceps, hamstrings, and the calf muscles and lower back muscles.

THE HUNDRED

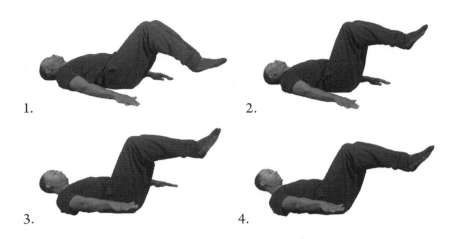

1.

2.

3.

4.

Step 1. Lie on your back.

Step 2. Your head and shoulders should be off the floor, knees slightly bent.

Step 3. Put your legs in a tabletop position (knees and hips should be at a ninety-degree angle). Keep your core (abdominal muscles) tight while maintaining your back firm on the floor.

Step 4. With your arms on each side, start movements as if you were splashing water (keep your arms straight; slightly lift them from the floor and then return them to the floor). Inhale when you lift your arms and exhale when you lower your arms. Repeat until you reach one hundred seconds.

Do this two or three times.

The *hundred* exercise is a classic Pilates warm-up routine that strengthens and tones the abdominal muscles.

The Criss-Cross

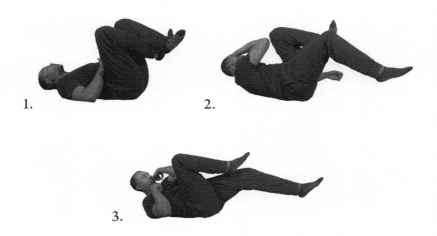

1.   2.

3.

Step 1. Lie on your back, tighten your abdominal muscles, and lift your legs off the floor. Keep your knees and hips at a ninety-degree angle.

Step 2. Lift your head and shoulders off the floor and inhale. Rotate the torso to the left. Use your right elbow to touch your left knee. Exhale and extend your left leg. Now inhale and rotate the torso to the right, using your left elbow to touch your right knee. Exhale and extend your right leg. Now repeat these movements and remember to breathe. This routine is done exactly like bicycles but with the movement of your arms.

Do fifteen to twenty repetitions, three sets.

The *criss-cross* exercise strengthens the abdominal muscles with special emphasis on the obliques. This routine also increases the flexibility of the spine.

BRIDGE

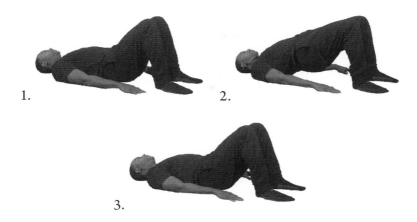

Step 1. Lie on your back. Bend your knees. Keep your feet flat on the floor.

Step 2. Raise your hips off the floor. Tighten your gluteal muscles and inhale. Your body should form a straight line from your shoulders to your knees. Pause at the top for a few seconds.

Step 3. Slowly lower your body and exhale.

Do fifteen to twenty repetitions.

The *bridge* or *hip raise* is an excellent exercise to strengthen and tone your bottom, calf muscles, and the core. Some target muscles that are emphasized in the routine are the hip adductors, the gluteus maximus, the hamstrings, the quadriceps, and the rectus abdominis.

SHOULDER STRETCH

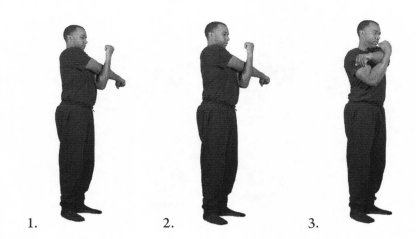

1.   2.   3.

Step 1. Stand with your feet shoulder-width apart, chest up, and head back over your shoulders. Now simply bring your right arm across your body.

Step 2. With your left arm, push against the right elbow. Then switch to the opposite arm. Hold fifteen seconds and repeat on the opposite side.

Do fifteen repetitions.

The *shoulder stretch* exercise should be performed if you have healthy shoulders. Some of the target muscles that are strengthened are the deltoid, pectoralis, and trapezius muscles.

TRICEPS STRETCH

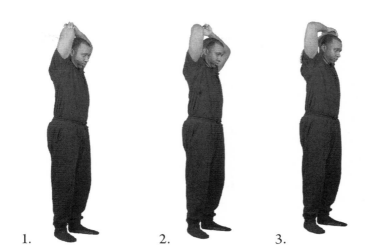

1.   2.   3.

Step 1. Simply bring your right arm up above and back. Bend your elbow.

Step 2. With your left hand up and over your head, push your right elbow back toward the middle of your back.

Step 3. Repeat with the opposite arm. Hold for fifteen seconds.

Do fifteen stretches on each side.

The *triceps stretch* exercise strengthens the triceps and increases the flexibility of the shoulder joints.

FOREARM STRETCH

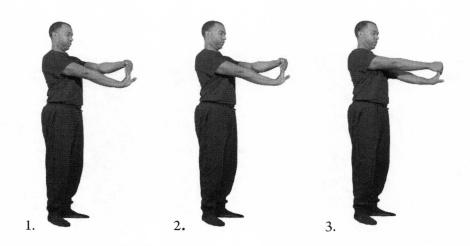

1.   2.   3.

Step 1. Extend your right arm in front of you with the palm up.

Step 2. Place your left hand over your right fingers and press toward you. Hold five seconds.

Do fifteen stretches on each forearm.

CORKSCREW

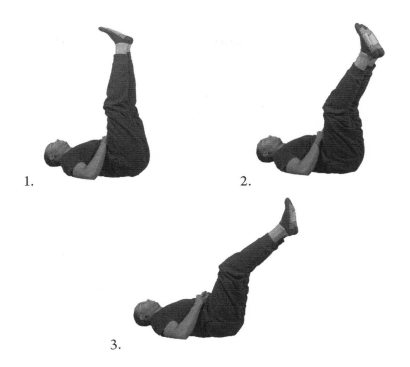

1.

2.

3.

Step 1. Lie on your back with both legs straight up toward the ceiling.

Step 2. Slowly move your legs to the right in a rotating motion, like you are making a big letter D. Inhale as you elevate your legs and then exhale as you lower your legs and rotate.

Step 3. Rotate to the left, creating the same letter D but backward.

Do ten repetitions, three sets.

The benefits of this exercise are core control, shoulder stability, and abdominal muscle strengthening.

Caution—avoid if you have neck or lower-back problems.

SINGLE LEG LIFT

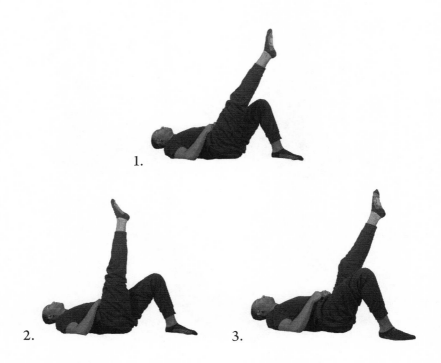

Step 1. Lie on your back, tighten your abdominal muscles, and bend your left knee with your foot on the floor.

Step 2. Keeping the knee extended, lift the right leg until the hip is close to a ninety-degree angle; then slowly lower the leg. Inhale as you lift the leg and exhale as you lower the leg. Inhale and exhale as you change legs.

Step 3. Now flex the right knee. Inhale and tighten the abdominal muscles, and repeat the movement, elevating the left leg.

Do ten repetitions, three sets.

The *single leg lift* exercise strengthens the abdominal muscles as well as those of the lower extremities.

Double Leg Lift

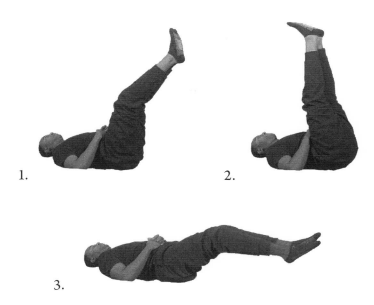

1.

2.

3.

Step 1. Lie on your back and engage your core by tightening the abdominal muscles.

Step 2. Raise both legs at the same time, keeping your knees straight and hips at a ninety-degree angle. Inhale as you raise your legs.

Step 3. Lower your legs slowly, almost touching the floor, and then raise both legs up again. Exhale as you lower the legs and inhale as you raise them.

Do ten repetitions, three sets.

The *double leg lift* exercise can be performed only if you have a healthy back. Some of the target muscles of this routine are the abdominal muscles, quadriceps, hamstrings, and muscles of the lower back.

STEP UP WITH KICK-BACK

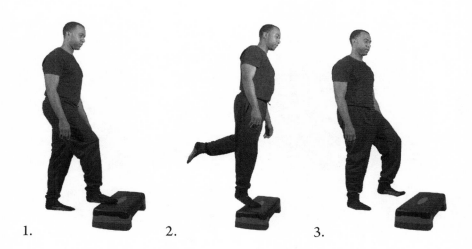

1.   2.   3.

Step 1. Using a step or wooden box, simply step onto the step with one foot.

Step 2. Kick back with the opposite leg, squeezing the gluteal muscles.

Step 3. Step down, switch to the opposite leg, and do the same thing.

Do this exercise for fifteen to twenty repetitions, three sets.

This exercise routine strengthens and tones the gluteal muscles as well as the muscles of the legs.

Be cautious if you do not have healthy knees.

Bulgarian Split Squat

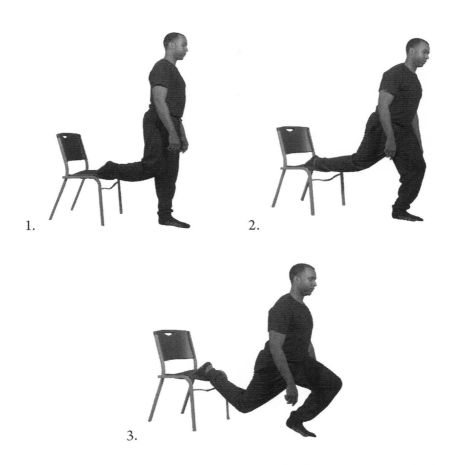

Step 1. Face away from a step chair or wooden box. Rest your right foot on this object while maintaining your weight on your left leg.

Step 2. Lower your hips, keeping your core tight and torso erect. Bend the left knee and continue to lower your hips until the right knee almost touches the floor.

Step 3. With the right foot still firmly planted on top of the chair or box, gently raise your body up to a standing position. Repeat twenty times.

Step 4. Switch to the opposite leg and do the same exercise. Repeat twenty times.

The *Bulgarian split squat* exercise targets the muscles of the lower body and abdominals.

Cautions—this routine should be done only if you have healthy knees and hips.

ELEVATED BRIDGE

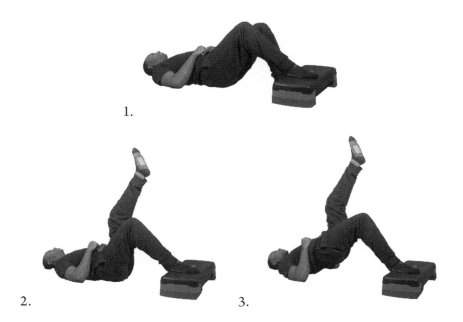

1.

2.

3.

Step 1. Lie down on your back.

Step 2. Use the step, chair, or wooden box. Rest one foot on the object of choice, bending the knee. The other leg should be straight up in the air.

Step 3. Push yourself up from the floor, using your upper back and heel. Be sure to tighten the gluteus muscles while keeping the core engaged. Now repeat the routine using the other leg.

Do fifteen to twenty repetitions, three sets.

This is another full-body workout routine, which targets muscles like the gluteus group and quadriceps.

Caution—perform only if you have a healthy back.

CRUNCH

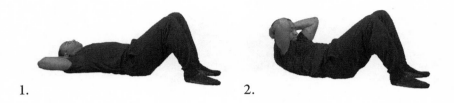

1.   2.

Step 1. Lie down on your back with both knees slightly bent.

Step 2. With your arms behind your head or crossed over your chest, raise your head (do not pull on your neck) and shoulders off the floor while tightening your abdominal muscles.

Do fifteen to twenty repetitions, three sets.

Crunches are a classic exercise for the muscles of the abdomen but also place tension on the lower back.

SUPERMAN

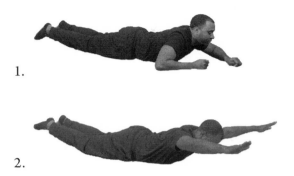

1.

2.

Step 1. Lie facedown. To begin, you need to be flat on your stomach on the floor facing toward the floor.

Step 2. Extend both arms in front of you with palms facing the floor. Now lift your arms and legs at the same time as if you were flying. Keep your core stationary.

Do fifteen to twenty repetitions, three sets.

The *superman* exercise routine works the muscles of the back as well as those of the upper and lower body. Some of the target muscles are the erector spinae, gluteus maximus, hamstring, deltoid, and trapezius muscles.

Caution—do only if you have a healthy back. You need to do a warm-up routine before performing this exercise. Start slowly.

RUNNING IN PLACE

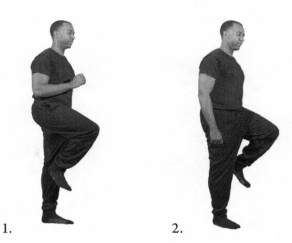

1.   2.

Step 1. While standing, lift one knee at a time. Begin to run in place. Increase speed gradually until you achieve a desirable speed.

Do this for three to five minutes.

Running in place engages the muscles of the entire body and increases the flexibility of the knees, hips, elbows, and shoulders.

SQUATS WITH A TWIST

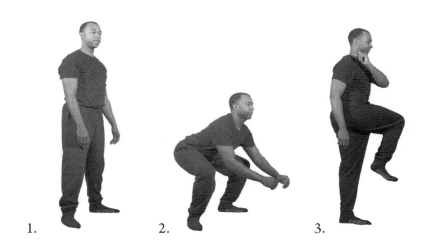

1.   2.   3.

Step 1. Stand with your feet shoulder-width apart.

Step 2. Squat down.

Step 3. Then stand back up into starting position and bring your right knee up. Slightly twist your body and touch your left elbow to your right knee.

Step 4. Repeat steps 1 and 2 again but with the other leg.

Do fifteen to twenty repetitions, three sets.

This is a full-body workout routine. The target muscles are the deep back muscles, obliques, quadriceps, and gluteus muscle group.

SQUAT ON CHAIR

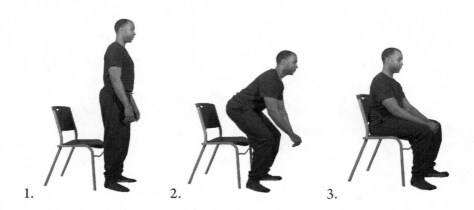

1.　　　　2.　　　　3.

Step 1. Stand upright with your feet shoulder-width apart, facing away from a chair.

Step 2. Slowly sit on the chair. Tighten your abdominal muscles. Keep the core engaged as you slowly return to a standing position. (Do not use your hands for support.)

Do fifteen to twenty repetitions, three sets.

The *squat on chair* routine strengthens and tones the muscles of the lower body, from the gluteus muscle group to those of the ankles. Strengthening these muscles gives stability to the lower extremities, thus preventing falls, especially in the elderly.

KNEE EXTENSION

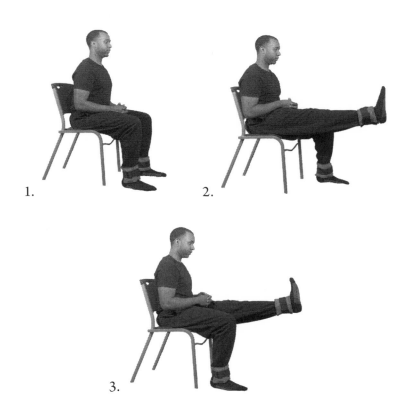

Step 1. Sit on a chair with your back supported. You can use three- to five-pound ankle weights. Place your hands on your thighs. Extend one leg until the knee is straight and the leg is parallel to the floor. Hold in position for two to three seconds. Now flex your foot with your toes pointing to your head. Hold in that position for two to three seconds.

Step 2. Bring the leg back to a ninety-degree angle flexed position with your feet on the floor.

Step 3. Repeat this exercise with the opposite leg. Alternate legs until you have done the exercise fifteen to twenty times.

Do six to eight sets.

The *knee extension* exercise strengthens and tones the thigh muscles and quadriceps and increases the strength and flexibility of the knee. If you have had knee surgery or pain, you can perform this routine without the ankle weights.

Hip Abduction

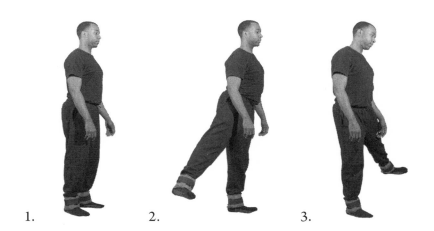

1.   2.   3.

Step 1. In a standing position, keep your body upright. You may use a chair for support.

Step 2. With ankle weights in place, simply raise one leg to the side away from your body.

Step 3. Now bring that leg back in toward the other leg. Repeat these movements twenty to thirty times. Now change to the other leg and repeat.

Do twenty to thirty repetitions, six sets.

This routine strengthens the gluteus muscles as well as the lateral hip muscles in order to improve hip stability, especially when engaging in lateral movements, such as turning.

STANDING LEG CURL

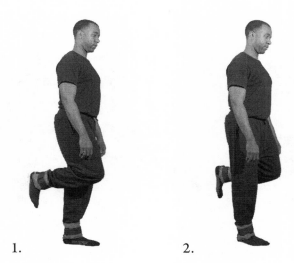

1.   2.

Step 1. Stand upright and tighten your abdominal muscles, maintaining your balance. You may support yourself with your hands on your hips or on a chair. Now bend or flex your knee. Then extend the knee. Repeat these extension and flexion movements twenty to thirty times and then place the leg back on the floor.

Step 2. Repeat with the other leg.

Do six sets.

This exercise strengthens and defines the hamstrings and the quadriceps and increases the flexibility of the knees.

PART 4

Eat to Beat and Treat

CHAPTER 16

Amazing Meal Plans and Recipes Guide

In this section, I have put together recipes that I have used with hundreds of my patients over the past several years. These patients, some of whom you have met as you read this book, are doing well. Many have lost weight, improved or reversed their disease processes, and are enjoying optimal health.

The recipes are simple and easy to prepare; however, for maximum benefit and to ensure that you adhere to the program, I advise you to plan and prepare your meals in advance. You will notice that the recipes have no animal fats and are mostly prepared from whole-grain, plant-based foods. Feel free to modify these recipes if you desire and as you become more confident and experienced, do not hesitate to create new recipes with foods that you and your family will enjoy for life.

At this point, I believe that you will agree with Hippocrates's statement, "Let food be thy medicine and medicine be thy food." Poor food choices can also be the most important disease-causing agent. So I applaud you for your desire to take charge of your health as your begin this journey to a long, happy life and amazing health. For more recipes, visit my website (www.cooperwellnesscenter.com) and be on the lookout for my cookbook.

Fourteen-Day Kick-Start to Amazing Health Meal Plans

Week 1

- cashew oat waffle
- quinoa salad
- garden minestrone soup
- Dr. Cooper's oats on the go
- walnut balls
- white beans and kale soup
- curried white bean spread
- tabbouleh
- lentil soup
- heart-healthy bean chili
- chickpea curry
- Jamaican red pea soup
- roasted vegetables with tofu
- mashed cauliflower and white beans
- baked eggplant and zucchini
- hummus
- blueberry whole wheat pancake
- cream of pumpkin soup

Week 2

- bean burritos
- Dr. Cooper's granola
- lentil burger
- French toast
- avocado vegetable wrap
- zucchini cauliflower soup
- whole wheat waffle
- brown rice and black bean salad
- tofu eggless salad

- cold summer soup
- scrambled tofu with kale
- chiles rellenos
- chickpea avocado spread
- Jamaican stewed peas
- Chinese stir-fry
- pasta primavera
- spinach kale soup

Amazing Health Recipes

Banana Whole Wheat Muffin

This is a great breakfast option, but eat with moderation if you are diabetic.

- 1 3/4 cups whole wheat flour
- 2 teaspoons baking soda
- 1/4 teaspoon salt
- 1/4 teaspoon ground nutmeg
- 2/3 cup crushed pineapple
- 2/3 cup almond milk
- 1/2 cup mashed very ripe banana
- 1 teaspoon vanilla
- 1/2 cup raisins
- 1/4 cup chopped pecans

Preheat oven to 400 degrees Fahrenheit. Line 12 standard muffin cups with paper baking cups or grease bottoms. Stir together whole wheat flour, baking soda, salt, and nutmeg in a medium bowl. Mix crushed pineapple, milk, banana and vanilla in a large bowl. Stir in the flour mixture just until moistened (batter will be lumpy). Fold in raisins and pecans. Divide batter evenly among muffin cups. Bake 18 to 20 minutes or until golden brown and a toothpick inserted into the center comes out clean. Remove from pan to wire rack. Serve warm.

Oven Roasted Potatoes

This is a great side dish you can enjoy any time of the day. You could also add firm tofu (cubes) and bake. Makes a great main dish.

- 4 pounds small red potatoes, halved

1 1/2 tablespoon olive oil

4 teaspoons fresh rosemary, chopped

2 teaspoons Mrs. Dash seasoning

1 medium onion, chopped

2 tablespoons McKay's seasoning

1 teaspoon salt, to taste

Preheat oven to 400 degrees Fahrenheit. Place potatoes in a single-layer baking sheet and sprinkle oil over potatoes. Then evenly mix in all the other ingredients. Cover with foil and bake for 12 to 15 minutes. Remove foil and continue to bake for an additional 15 minutes or until golden brown.

Bean Burrito

This is a well-known and easy-to-prepare Mexican dish. These can be served at any time of the day.

1 whole wheat tortilla

1/4 cup spicy Mexican beans (mashed)

desired amount of:

chopped lettuce

chopped tomatoes

diced onions

olives

avocado

salsa

soy sour cream (or Wayfare Food brand)

Warm tortillas and spread the beans over the tortillas. Fold like an envelope. Serve with lettuce, tomato, onions, olives, and avocado and top with salsa and soy sour cream.

Scramble Tofu with Kale

This great dish is filled with lots of vitamins, antioxidants, protein, fiber, and phytochemicals.

> 1 (16-ounce) water-packed package of extra-firm organic tofu
> 2 teaspoons vegetable oil
> 1/2 cup chopped onion
> 1/4 cup bell peppers
> 2 teaspoons savory seasoning
> 1/2 teaspoon turmeric powder
> 1/2 teaspoon salt
> 1/2 teaspoon onion powder
> 1/2 teaspoon garlic powder
> 1/2 teaspoon thyme
> 2 teaspoons Mrs. Dash
> 1/2 cup tomatoes
> 4 cups kale, coarsely chopped

Remove the tofu from its package, rinse, drain, and set aside. In a large skillet or saucepan, sauté in hot oil the onion, peppers, and spices for 5 minutes. Scramble tofu in skillet and add remaining ingredients except kale. Allow to cook for 7 minutes on medium heat. Add kale. Stir occasionally. Cover until kale is wilted, about another 3 to 5 minutes. Serve with whole wheat bread or baked potatoes or over brown rice (main dish).

Traditional Tofu Scramble

This dish looks and taste like eggs but without the cholesterol. It is even more delicious when left overnight in the refrigerator.

> 1 (16-ounce) water-packed package of extra-firm organic tofu

2 teaspoons vegetable oil

1/2 cup chopped onion

1/4 cup bell peppers

2 teaspoons McKay's savory seasoning

1/2 teaspoon turmeric powder

1/2 teaspoon salt

1/2 teaspoon onion powder

1/2 teaspoon garlic powder

1/2 teaspoon thyme

1 teaspoon Mrs. Dash

1/2 cup tomatoes

Remove the tofu from its package, rinse, drain, and set aside. In large skillet/saucepan sauté in hot oil the onion, peppers, and spices for 5 minutes. Scramble tofu in the skillet and add the remaining ingredients. Cover and allow to cook for another 10 minutes. Serve as filling for tacos or with whole wheat bread.

Whole Wheat Pancakes

These delicious pancakes will not raise your cholesterol.

3 cups whole wheat flour

2 1/2 teaspoons baking powder

1/2 teaspoon salt

2 cups soy milk

3 tablespoons applesauce

Mix dry ingredients together. Add remaining ingredients and mix well gently. Drop mixture by spoonful on a hot, nonstick griddle. Fry until golden brown. Flip pancake and repeat for the other side. Serve with fruit topping.

Cashew-Oat Waffle

These waffles are filling and great for people with heart disease, diabetes and high cholesterol. A diet high in fiber will promote better glucose and cholesterol levels. Serves 2 to 3.

> 1/3 cup raw cashews
> 2 cups water or 1 cup soy milk
> 1 teaspoon vanilla extract
> 2 cups old-fashioned oats
> 1/2 teaspoon salt

Blend cashews in water or soy milk until smooth. Add remaining ingredients, and then blend together. Let mixture stand 5 minutes to thicken. Cook approximately 7 minutes in the waffle iron until golden brown. Serve hot with your favorite fruit topping. Waffles freeze well and can be easily reheated in a toaster or microwave.

Mushroom and Kale Frittata

This simple dish is good for breakfast but could be eaten any time of the day. Store leftovers in the refrigerator and rewarm in the oven. Makes 6 servings.

> 1 cup rolled oats
> 1/2 cup whole wheat flour
> 1/2 teaspoon baking soda
> 1/4 teaspoon salt
> 1 cup soy milk
> 2 tablespoons olive oil
> 1 small onion, chopped
> 2 cups mushrooms
> 2 cups scrambled tofu (refer to recipe)

4 cups coarsely chopped kale leaves

2 cloves garlic, mashed and minced

Blend oats; add wheat flour, baking soda, and salt. In a separate bowl, mix milk and oil. Then combine both and set aside. Spray large ovenproof skillet with nonstick cooking spray, and heat over medium heat. Add onion and mushrooms; cook and stir 6 to 8 minutes or until onion is light golden. Add kale and garlic; cook 3 to 5 minutes or until kale is wilted. Evenly spread mixture to cover the bottom of the skillet. Pour scrambled tofu over the kale mixture. Cover and cook 6 to 7 minutes or until almost set. Poor batter mixture over sautéed vegetable tofu and slightly mix. Preheat broiler. Uncover skillet. Broil 2 to 3 minutes or until golden brown and set. Let stand 5 minutes before cutting into 6 wedges.

Baked Oats

This is an excellent breakfast dish and is filled with fiber and good fat, which are very filling and will eliminate the urge to snack.

2 cups rolled oats

1/4 cup raisins

1/4 cup dates, chopped

1 teaspoon ground cinnamon

1 teaspoon baking powder

1 cup soy or almond milk

1/2 cup blended apple

1 teaspoon vanilla extract

1/2 cup almond slivers

Mix all dry ingredients in a bowl, and then add the wet ingredients and mix well. Preheat oven to 350 degrees Fahrenheit. Place mixture in a lightly oiled baking dish, spread evenly, and cover and bake for 25 to 30 minutes. Serve warm or cold.

Strawberry Peach Smoothie

Smoothies are quick and easy to make. Keep small bags of frozen fruits and vegetables handy.

    4 cups strawberries, frozen
    4 cups peaches, frozen
    2 tablespoons flax seeds
    1 cup vanilla almond milk

Place everything in a high-speed blender and blend until smooth.

Banana Berry Smoothie

    4 cups strawberries, frozen
    3 ripe bananas, frozen
    3 cups soy or almond milk
    1/2 cup rolled oats

Place everything in a high-speed blender and blend until smooth.

Green Smoothie

    2 cups kale
    2 cups romaine lettuce
    2 cups spinach
    1 green apple
    1 cup water

Place all the ingredients in a high-speed blender and blend until smooth.

Blueberry-Oatmeal Pancakes

These pancakes are a little denser, heartier, and more filling than the regular pancakes.

  2 flax eggs (2 tablespoons ground flaxseed + 6 tablespoons water)
  1 cup rolled oats
  1 1/2 cup unsweetened soy or almond milk
  1/4 cup walnuts
  1/2 cup whole wheat flour
  1/2 teaspoon baking soda
  1/2 teaspoon baking powder
  6 dates, pitted
  1/2 teaspoon salt
  1 cup fresh or frozen blueberries

Mix ground flax with 6 tablespoons of water and let mix stand for 10 minutes. The consistency should be that of an egg. Place oats, nuts, and milk in blender and blend until smooth. Place mixture in bowl, and then fold in other ingredients. Add more milk if necessary for the desired consistency. Lightly grease the hot skillet or pan with additional oil. Pour 1/2 cup pancake rounds on the skillet and cook until bubbles form on the surface. Carefully drop 6 to 8 (optional) blueberries onto one side of each pancake, and then flip and cook on the other side until golden brown.

French Toast

This is a healthier and delicious spin on the traditional fat-laden French toast.

  1 ripe banana
  1 cup unsweetened soy or almond milk
  2 tablespoons cornstarch

1/2 teaspoon pure vanilla extract
1/2 teaspoon nutmeg
tiny pinch of salt
6 slices whole wheat bread

Mash banana in a wide, shallow bowl. Mix in other ingredients, except the bread. Soak bread in the liquid mixture. Heat nonstick pan or griddle on medium heat and lightly spray with vegetable oil. Transfer the soaked bread to heated surface and cook until both sides are golden brown. Serve with fruit sauce or berries.

Huevos Rancheros

This great breakfast option is high in protein content and goes well with smashed cooked kidney beans.

1 1/2 teaspoons olive oil
1 (14- to 16-ounce package) firm tofu, drained and mashed with fork
1 medium onion, chopped
1 large clove garlic (mashed and minced)
1 medium green bell pepper, chopped
1 cup prepared medium or mild salsa, plus more for serving
2 medium tomatoes, diced (1 cup)
1–2 small fresh jalapeno chiles, seeded and minced
2 tablespoons nutritional yeast
2 teaspoons ground cumin
1/2 teaspoon ground turmeric
1 teaspoon Savory Seasoning powder
1 cup cilantro leaves, chopped
8 corn tortillas, warmed

Heat oil in large skillet over medium heat. Add onion and garlic and sauté 5 minutes or until translucent. Add bell pepper, crumbling each as it goes in. Stir in salsa, tomatoes, and chiles, followed by nutritional yeast (if using), cumin, savory seasoning, and turmeric. Cook 5 to 8 minutes or until tomatoes have softened and ingredients are melded. Stir in cilantro. Taste and add salt, if desired. Divide tofu mixture among tortillas, and serve with salsa.

Jamaican Cornmeal Porridge

This classical warm breakfast cereal is widely served in Jamaica. May add coconut cream for a creamier taste.

   1 cup yellow cornmeal
   4 cups water
   2 cinnamon sticks
   1/2 teaspoon salt
   1/2 teaspoon nutmeg
   1 cup soy or almond milk

Mix cornmeal in 1 cup water and set aside. Place 3 cups of water and cinnamon sticks in a deep, medium-sized pot. Bring water to a boil and then pour the cornmeal mixture into the boiling water. Turn heat down to low and stir continuously until thickened and smooth. Cover pot and allow to cook for 20 minutes. Add milk, salt, and nutmeg, and allow to cook for 10 minutes more. Sweeten to taste with natural sweetener, such as agave. Serve hot in a bowl.

Hot Bulgur Wheat Cereal

Delicious hearty breakfast ideal for diabetics because of the high fiber content but great for everyone.

   2 cups bulgur wheat
   4 cups almond or soy milk

2 cinnamon sticks

2 tablespoons whole wheat flour

1/2 teaspoon nutmeg

1/2 teaspoon salt (optional)

1/2 cup raisins

1/4 cup walnuts, chopped

1 ripe banana

Place bulgur wheat, cinnamon sticks, and milk in a deep, small- to medium-sized pot and allow to cook on low to medium heat for 25 minutes. Mix whole wheat flour in small amount of water and then pour this mixture into the pot. Stir and allow to cook for another 7 to 10 minutes more. Add nutmeg to mixture just before removing pot from heat. Serve hot in bowl topped with raisins, walnuts, and ripe banana to sweeten.

Toast and Gravy

If you are a lover of biscuits and gravy, then this breakfast option is for you. It is fast and easy to prepare, and most important, it is healthy with good fat.

1/2 cup almonds

2 cups water

2 tablespoons McKay's chicken-style seasoning

2 tablespoons Braggs amino soy

1 tablespoon nutritional yeast

1/2 teaspoon garlic powder

1/2 teaspoon onion powder

1 small onion

1/2 teaspoon dry basil

2 tablespoons cornstarch

Place all ingredients except cornstarch in a high-speed blender with 11/2 cup of water. Blend until smooth. Place mixture in a saucepan. Allow to simmer on medium heat. Mix cornstarch in remaining water and incorporate to boiling mixture. Stir frequently until smooth. Place toast bread on plate. Pour gravy over toast and enjoy!

Steamed Spinach

This dish is filled with vitamins, minerals, and antioxidants. You may use kale instead of spinach. Remember not to cook your vegetables, as this will destroy vital nutrients.

> 1 tablespoon olive oil
> 1/2 medium onion, chopped
> 1 small tomato, chopped
> 1/2 medium green bell pepper, chopped
> 2 (10-ounce) packages frozen spinach
> 2 sprigs fresh thyme
> 1 teaspoon McKay's chicken-style seasoning

Place oil in saucepan on low-medium heat. Sauté onion, bell pepper, and tomato for 3 to 5 minutes. Remove water from spinach and then add to saucepan. Add remaining ingredients. Allow to simmer for another 7 to 10 minutes. Taste and add extra seasoning or salt if desired. Serve with oven-roasted potatoes.

Granola

This recipe can be prepared on the weekend and then stored. You may serve with nondairy milk or consume dry as a snack. You could also add your favorite seeds and dried fruits. For diabetics, remember that dried fruits could raise your blood sugar, so limit your portion.

3 cups whole rolled oats

1/2 cup unsweetened coconut, shredded

1/2 cup almond slivers

1/2 cup wheat germ

1 cup raw sunflower seeds

1/2 cup sesame seeds, unsalted

3 cups banana, mashed

1/2 cup raisins

1/2 teaspoon salt

In a large bowl, mix together dry ingredients, except raisins, and then add the banana. Lightly oil-spray three baking sheets and then divide granola between the baking sheets and spread out evenly. Bake at 350 degrees Fahrenheit until golden brown. Stir every 5 minutes. Remove granola from oven and cool. Mix in raisins. Later, store granola in an airtight container to retain freshness.

Multigrain Waffles

Delicious and filling! These waffles can be made ahead, stored in the freezer, and warmed in a toaster when needed.

1/2 cup rolled oats

1/2 cup rye flour

1/2 cup whole wheat flour

1/2 cup soy flour

2 1/4 cups water or almond milk

1/2 teaspoon nutmeg

1 teaspoon cinnamon

2 tablespoons dates, chopped

1/2 teaspoon salt

Blend all ingredients until smooth. Let batter stand for 5 minutes to thicken. Blend again, and then pour onto a hot, slightly oiled waffle iron. Bake for 10 minutes. Serve hot with fruit topping.

Corn Bread

This is a tasty cornbread without the cholesterol from eggs or batter. Makes a great side dish.

>   1 package (10 ounces) soft tofu
>   1 cup cornmeal, uncooked
>   1 can cream-style corn
>   1 tablespoon olive oil
>   1 teaspoon baking soda
>   1 1/2 teaspoons baking powder
>   1/4 teaspoon clove or nutmeg, ground
>   1/2 teaspoon salt

Blend tofu, and then add all the other ingredients and continue blending until smooth. Pour batter into a slightly oil-sprayed 9-x-9-inch baking pan. Bake at 400 degrees Fahrenheit for 25 minutes or until golden brown. Allow to stand for a few minutes before serving.

Dr. Cooper's Oats-on-the-Go

This breakfast is quick and easy to prepare. It is filled with fiber to keep you satisfied all morning. It is also packed with protein, vitamins, and good fats.

>   1/2 cup old-fashioned oats
>   3/4 to 1 cup nondairy milk
>   1 ounce walnuts

1 ripe banana or 1/2 cup berries

1/4 teaspoon cinnamon

Place oats and milk in a microwavable bowl and microwave for 3 to 4 minutes. Carefully remove and top with banana slices or berries, nuts, and cinnamon. Enjoy!

MAIN MEALS

Heart-Healthy Bean Chili

This dish is a great meat substitute. It is high in protein and fiber. It is ideal for those who are losing weight and will keep your blood sugar down if you are diabetic. Serve with fresh mixed vegetables or with baked sweet potato.

    1 tablespoon olive oil or vegetable oil
    2 cups onions, diced
    4 cloves garlic, mashed and then minced
    1 cup carrots, chopped
    2 cups vegetable broth
    2 cups cooked kidney beans
    2 cups cooked red beans
    2 cups cooked black beans
    1 cup frozen corn
    3 cups cooked, chopped tomatoes
    3/4 cup of green bell pepper
    1 tablespoon cumin powder
    1 teaspoon dried oregano
    3–4 bay leaves
    1 teaspoon cayenne pepper
    1 teaspoon sea salt, to taste

In a large, deep pot, add vegetable/olive oil and sauté onions and garlic for 3 to 5 minutes. Then add vegetable broth and the remaining ingredients and spices. Allow the mixture to cook for another 20 minutes.

Hummus and Veggie Wrap

This dish is very quick and easy to prepare. There are different types of tortillas that you could use: sun-dried tomato, spinach, and whole wheat. You also have the option to add your favorite veggies.

> 2 (12-inch) whole-grain tortillas
> 1/2 cup hummus
> 1 cup spinach or kale
> 1 medium zucchini, cut in strips
> 1 large carrot, cut in strips
> 1/4 cup black olives
> 1/2 cup tomato, sliced
> 1/2 cup avocado, sliced
> 1/2 cucumber, sliced

Microwave the tortilla for a few seconds to make it pliable. Spread the hummus over the tortilla, and then layer on the assorted vegetables. Wrap the tortilla like a burrito and enjoy.

Tofu Thai Curry

My patients at the wellness center love this dish. It is delicious and very easy to prepare and goes well with brown rice. Store leftover in the refrigerator. The dish is even more delicious 1 to 3 days after. Be careful not to overeat. This is a high-fat dish.

> 1 (16-ounce) package of extra firm tofu, drained
> 1 tablespoon extra-virgin olive oil
> 1 medium onion, chopped
> 1 tablespoon garlic, mashed and minced
> 1 cup potatoes, cut in 1/2-inch cubes
> 1/2 cup carrots, cut in 1/2-inch cubes

1/2 cup yellow or red bell pepper, julienned

1/2 cup fresh or frozen peas

1 teaspoon ground cumin

8 fresh basil leaves, chopped, or 1/2 teaspoon dry basil

1 tablespoon ginger, minced finely

1 teaspoon curry powder

1 teaspoon turmeric powder

1 (14-ounce) can coconut milk

1 1/2 teaspoon salt or to taste

Preheat oven to 375 degrees Fahrenheit to begin baking the tofu. Spray a baking sheet with oil. Lay the tofu cubes out evenly and spray with oil. Then sprinkle with salt. Bake for about 20 minutes until golden brown. While the tofu is baking, prepare the curry. In a pot, sauté the onions, garlic, and other veggies over medium heat in olive oil until onions are transparent. Add ginger, curry powder, and turmeric. Then add coconut milk. Now incorporate tofu as well as all the other ingredients, cover, and allow to cook for 25 minutes or until veggies are cooked. Taste and add extra seasonings or salt. Enjoy!

Caribbean Curried Tofu

My daughter enjoys preparing this dish for large social or church events. Adding scotch bonnet pepper to this dish will give it the authentic Jamaican taste! Goes great with brown rice, roti, naan, or fresh mixed vegetables.

1 tablespoon vegetable oil

1 (12-ounce) package extra-firm tofu, drained and cubed

1 medium onion, chopped

4 cloves garlic, mashed and minced

2 teaspoons curry powder

1 teaspoon turmeric powder

1 tablespoon savory seasoning

1/2 cup carrots, sliced

1/2 cup potato, cubed

4 sprigs fresh thyme

1/4 cup green onion, chopped

1 (14-ounce can) coconut milk

1 teaspoon Mrs. Dash

1/2 teaspoon salt or to taste

Heat oil in large skillet or wok over medium-high heat. Add tofu and braze until golden brown on all sides, stirring intermittently for about 10 to 15 minutes. Remove and set aside. Lower heat to low-medium. Then add garlic and onion and sauté for 2 minutes. Then incorporate coconut milk, turmeric, curry, and the other ingredients. Return tofu to the skillet or wok. Allow it to cook for 15 to 20 minutes or until the carrots are tender. Taste and add extra spice if needed.

Hummus

Use as a dip for vegetables, pita, or multigrain chips. You may add vegetables, such as celery or bell pepper. This is a great party dish. Everyone enjoys hummus!

1/4 cup onion, chopped

2 cloves garlic, mashed and then minced

2 cups garbanzo beans, cooked

1/4 cup lemon juice

1/3 cup tahini

1/2 cup water

1/2 teaspoon salt

1 tablespoon cumin

1/2 cup roasted bell pepper

On low heat sauté onion and garlic, using a small amount of water. Then combine all ingredients in a food processor or high-speed blender and blend until smooth. Add water as needed. Taste and add more seasonings if desired.

Black Bean Burger

This is a great burger to replace meat, which is high in saturated fat. If you want to keep your cholesterol down, then this is a great alternative for a healthy lunch meal.

> 1 (15-ounce) can black beans, drained
> 1/2 jalapeno, seeded and chopped
> 3 garlic cloves
> 1/2 medium onion, cut in wedges
> 2/3 cup rolled oats
> 1/2 cup frozen corn
> 1 tablespoon fresh cilantro, minced
> 2 teaspoon ground cumin
> 1/2 teaspoon curry powder
> 1/4 teaspoon cayenne pepper
> 1/4 cup bread crumbs
> 1/2 teaspoon salt or more to taste
> tomato
> mustard
> ketchup

In a medium bowl, mash beans with fork and set aside. Place the onion, jalapeno, and garlic in a food processor and pulse 5 to 6 times. Add oats, corn, cilantro, cumin, curry powder, and cayenne. Season to taste with salt, and pulse about 10 to 12 times. Remove ingredients from food processor and add to bowl with mashed beans and stir well. Spray a small amount of oil into a skillet and heat to medium. Form the burger mixture into 4 equal patties. Cook the patties for 5 to 7 minutes on each side or until a golden crust develops and the patties are heated through. Remove the patties from the heat and place onto burger buns. Add sliced tomato, lettuce, mustard, and ketchup.

Baked Falafel

Falafel is a well-known vegetarian dish that is served in a pita bread pocket with hummus and fresh vegetables. Feel free to add your special spices and herbs.

> 1 1/2 (15-ounce) can garbanzo beans (chickpeas), drained, and 1/4 cup liquid reserved
> 1/4 cup fresh lemon juice
> 1 small onion, finely chopped
> 2 cloves garlic
> 1/4 cup fresh cilantro
> 1/2 teaspoon dried basil
> 1/2 teaspoon dried oregano
> 1 teaspoon cumin
> 1/4 teaspoon cayenne
> 1/2 teaspoon paprika
> 1 teaspoon salt
> 1 1/2 cups whole wheat bread crumbs

Preheat the oven to 350 degrees Fahrenheit. In a food processor, add the garbanzo beans, fresh lemon juice, onion, and garlic, and puree until smooth. Put the bean mixture in a large bowl and add all the other dry seasoning (oregano, basil, cumin, cayenne, paprika, and salt). Then, stir in the bread crumbs to hold the mixture together. Add more bread crumbs if the mixture is not holding together. Roll into 1-inch balls, and place them on a cooking sheet. Lightly spray the falafel with oil and bake in the oven for 10 to 15 minutes per side or until falafel are lightly browned. Test for doneness by pressing the outside with your finger. The falafel should come out moist inside and give to the pressure of your finger.

Tofu "Egg" Salad

This dish is very simple and easy to prepare. Feel free to add other vegetables and spices, such as bell pepper and shredded carrots. Serve as a spread on bread or stuff into pita bread.

> 1 pounds firm tofu, drained and crumbled
> 1/4 cup vegenaise
> 2 tablespoons prepared mustard
> 1/2 teaspoon ground turmeric
> 1 tablespoon soy sauce
> 1 teaspoon onion powder
> 1 teaspoon garlic powder
> 3 to 4 scallions, finely chopped
> 1/4 cup minced celery

Place the tofu in a bowl and mash with a potato masher. Add the vegenaise (if desired), mustard, soy sauce, and turmeric. Mix well until the tofu takes on a bright-yellow color. Stir in the scallions, celery, and relish, if desired. Chill for an hour or more before serving.

Curried Bean Sandwich Spread

This dish is very versatile. You can use it as a sandwich spread, stuffing for pita bread, or dip for your favorite veggies. Great dish for a social event.

> 3/4 cup water
> 1 onion, finely chopped
> 1 green bell pepper, diced
> 1/2 cup diced carrots

2 cloves garlic, mashed and then minced

1 teaspoon curry powder

1 teaspoon ground cumin

1/2 teaspoon thyme, dried

1 tablespoon savory seasoning (McKay chicken-style seasoning)

3 cups cooked white beans

Add water and vegetables to saucepan. Cook for 10 minutes. Then add all other ingredients, including curry power, turmeric, savory seasoning, and beans. Allow to cook for 12 to 15 minutes. Stir occasionally. Taste and add more seasoning as desired. Remove from the heat. Allow to cook. Then puree in a food processor. Enjoy!

Coconut Curry Chickpea

Chickpeas (garbanzo beans) are very high in fiber and a great protein source and can be used in many different menus. This dish can be enjoyed with baked sweet potato, brown (wild) rice, mixed steamed vegetables. It can also be pureed and served as a sandwich spread or as a dip.

1 cup coconut milk

2 teaspoons curry powder

2 teaspoons turmeric

1/2 cup chopped onions

2 cloves garlic, mashed and chopped

1 teaspoon thyme

1 teaspoon cumin

2 teaspoons savory seasoning salt

1 teaspoon sea salt (or to taste)

2 (15-ounce) cans chickpeas

1 small potato (cubed)

a dash of scotch bonnet or cayenne pepper (optional)

In a large, deep pot, first sauté a small amount of coconut milk, curry, and turmeric. Allow it to simmer for 2 to 3 minutes on low-medium heat. Then add onion and garlic, thyme, and other spices. Add potato and chickpeas. Add remaining portion of coconut milk and allow to simmer on low-medium heat for another 30 minutes or until potato is tender.

Coconut Curry Eggplant

This is a great dish, simple and easy to prepare. It goes well with steamed, mixed veggies. It can also be pureed and served with whole wheat pasta.

1/2 cup coconut milk
2 teaspoons turmeric powder
2 teaspoons curry powder
1 medium onion, chopped
3 cloves of garlic, mashed and diced
1 medium green bell pepper, diced
2 large eggplants, cut in large cubes
1 teaspoon thyme
2 teaspoons savory seasoning salt
1 teaspoon salt, to taste

Sauté curry powder and turmeric in coconut milk on low heat for 1 to 2 minutes. Then add onion, garlic, and bell pepper and simmer for another 2 minutes. Then add eggplant and the remaining ingredients. Allow to cook on low medium heat for 30 minutes or until cooked. May serve with cooked brown rice or may blend and use as a sauce, which may be poured over cooked pasta.

Seasoned Oven Fries

Healthy replacement for French fries—tasty and delicious without the oil!

    4 large potatoes
    1 teaspoon Mrs. Dash
    1 tablespoon McKay's seasoning
    2 tablespoons soy sauce

Thinly slice the potatoes lengthwise. Place the potatoes in a flat baking dish. Mix all the other ingredients together then pour over the potatoes and marinate for 1 hour, turning occasionally to make sure that all are coated. Preheat oven to 450 degrees Fahrenheit. Place the potatoes on a nonstick baking sheet. Bake for 45 minutes or until lightly browned, basting occasionally with dressing.

Roasted Vegetable Delight

This quick and easy recipe can be enjoyed at any meal. Leftovers are even more delicious.

    1 zucchini, green
    1 zucchini, yellow
    3 cups broccoli
    3 cups cauliflower
    1 cup carrots
    1 cup red pepper
    1/2 cup diced onion
    8 ounces of firm tofu
    2 tablespoons Braggs amino or soy sauce
    1 package Lipton onion soup mix

All vegetables and tofu should be cut into small bite-sized pieces. Mix together all the ingredients in a large baking dish, cover, and bake at 400 degrees Fahrenheit for 10 minutes. Open and mix ingredients together. Then bake for another 10 to 15 minutes.

Chiles Rellenos

This Mexican dish is delicious. The filling can be made with your favorite vegetables and spices.

olive-oil spray
1 large onion, finely chopped
3 cloves garlic, mashed and then minced
1 large green bell pepper, finely chopped
1 cup water
4 cups brown rice, cooked
6 cups mixed vegetables (frozen corn, peas, carrots)
2 small zucchini, finely chopped
1 (8-ounce) can tomato sauce
2 teaspoons dried Mexican oregano
2 teaspoons ground cumin
10 small roasted poblano chiles, peeled, deveined
2 cups of soy veggie crumbles
shredded veggie cheese

Heat oven to 350 degrees Fahrenheit. Spray oil in large skillet and heat on medium-high heat. Add onions, garlic, and bell pepper, stirring frequently, and allow to cook for 4 to 5 minutes. Add vegetables and a small amount of water. Then allow the mixture to cook for another 10 minutes. Add tomato sauce, seasoning, and vegetarian crumbles, cover, and allow to cook for 5 to 7 minutes. Taste and add more spices if needed. Spoon into chile; place in shallow baking dish. Cover. Bake 20 minutes. Top with shredded cheese. Bake, uncovered, 5 minutes or until melted.

Oats Walnut Balls

These no-meat meatballs are packed with fiber and protein while low in fat. You can add your special gravy, but it also goes well with marinara sauce.

  4 cups water
  1 cup chopped walnuts
  1 cup chopped sunflower seeds
  1/2 cup Braggs amino acid or soy sauce
  2 tablespoons olive oil (optional)
  1/4 cup nutritional yeast flakes
  1 teaspoon garlic powder
  2 teaspoons onion powder
  2 cloves garlic, mashed and diced
  1 medium onion, chopped
  1 tablespoon dried basil
  1 teaspoon thyme
  1 teaspoon ground coriander
  1 teaspoon sage
  4 cups rolled oats

Pour water in pot. Add all ingredients except rolled oats. Bring to a boil and then stir in rolled oats and cover. Remove from heat, cover, and set aside. When mixture is cooled, form 3-inch patties 1 1/2 inch thick (form into balls). Place on oiled baking sheet and bake on each side for 15 minutes at 350 to 400 degrees Fahrenheit. Enjoy with your own sauce. Can be served with spaghetti.

Dr. Cooper's Rosemary-Lemon Tofu Kabobs

These are absolutely delicious, without the danger of saturated fat from beef or chicken. A great dish for parties or any social events.

4 small red potatoes, quartered

1 pack tofu cut in squares

1/8 teaspoon Stubbs beef-like seasoning

1 yellow onion

1/2 teaspoon dried rosemary

dash of paprika

1 red bell pepper

2 tablespoons lemon juice

1 tablespoon olive oil

1 teaspoon grated lemon peel

1/2 clove garlic, minced

1/2 teaspoon salt

Preheat broiler. Steam potatoes 6 minutes or until crisp to tender. Rinse under cold water. Dry with paper towels. Sprinkle tofu evenly with Stubbs beef-like seasoning. Thread potatoes into 4 (10-inch) metal skewers, alternating with tofu and onion. Spray lightly with nonstick cooking spray. Sprinkle with rosemary and paprika. Place kabobs on baking sheet; broil 4 minutes. Turn over, and broil 4 more or until tofu is brown. Meanwhile, combine remaining ingredients in a small bowl. Spoon lemon mixture evenly over kabobs.

Jamaican Stewed Peas

This dish is high in protein and fiber and goes well with rice, potatoes, or steamed mixed veggies. A great dish for diabetics, the high fiber content promotes blood sugar control.

2 cups dry red kidney beans

1 large onion, chopped

2 stalks scallion, mashed and chopped

4 cloves garlic

3 sprigs fresh thyme, chopped

2 teaspoons savory seasoning salt

1 (15-ounce) can coconut milk

2 tablespoons vegetable or olive oil

Place beans in 8 cups water and soak overnight. Pour water off. Add 6 cups water and cook for about 2 hours until tender. Add all the other ingredients and allow to simmer on low-medium heat for 1 hour until cooked. Serve with seasoned brown rice and fresh vegetable salad.

Cashew Brown Rice Loaf

This is quick and easy to prepare. Serve with cashew or mushroom gravy on a bed of green vegetable salad.

1 cup cashews, raw

2 cups steamed brown rice

2 cups rich nut or soy milk

2 large onions, chopped

1 cup celery, finely chopped

4 slices of bread, crumbled

2 teaspoon Braggs amino or soy

2 tablespoons thyme

2 teaspoons sage

1 teaspoon celery seed

1 teaspoon salt or to taste

Place nuts in food processor and chop. Add all other ingredients and continue to process. Spoon into baking dish. Cover and place dish in pan of water. Bake 1 hour at 350 degrees Fahrenheit.

Bean Burrito

This is a common Mexican dish that is packed with protein and fiber. Feel free to add other fillings, such as black beans or sautéed vegetables and cabbage.

> whole grain tortillas
> spicy Mexican beans or mashed cooked pinto beans
> salsa—fresh tomato or healthy ketchup
> avocado slices
> cucumber slices
> green leaf lettuce

Warm tortillas in oven or skillet to soften. Spread lightly with cashew cheese sauce or other soy mayonnaise. Spoon 1/3 to 1/2 cup bean filling onto each tortilla. Top with salsa, sliced avocado, cucumber, and green lettuce. Garnish with parsley and green onion curls. Serve with crisp cabbage coleslaw and your favorite soup for a complete meal.

Oat-Nut Burgers

This burger patty is filled with fiber and good fat. Serve with tomato and lettuce on whole wheat bun or bread.

> 2 cups rolled oats
> 1/2 teaspoon onion powder
> 1 cup finely chopped walnuts
> 1/2 teaspoon coriander
> 1/2 teaspoon sage
> 1 tablespoon soy sauce
> 1/2 teaspoon garlic powder
> 1/2 teaspoon dried sage
> 1 small onion, finely chopped

2 cups hot water

1 tablespoon nutritional yeast

Place all the ingredients in hot water, cover, and let rest for 20 minutes. Form into six or eight patties. Cook on a nonstick griddle over medium heat until browned on each side, 20 to 30 minutes.

Spicy Tofu Burgers

These burgers are tasty, high in protein, and low in calories, so enjoy!

1 pound firm tofu, drained

2 cups rolled oats

2 tablespoons soy sauce

1 tablespoon cumin

1 tablespoon chili powder

1/2 teaspoon Mrs. Dash or Italian herbs

1 teaspoon garlic powder

1 teaspoon onion powder

1 teaspoon grated fresh ginger

1 small onion, finely chopped

2 tablespoons fresh thyme, finely chopped or minced

Preheat the oven to 350 degrees Fahrenheit. Place the tofu in a large bowl and mash with a potato masher. Add the remaining ingredients and stir until well combined. Moisten your hands. Shape into eight patties and place on a nonstick baking sheet. Bake for 20 minutes on the first side; turn over and bake an additional 10 minutes. May also cook on stovetop using a slightly oiled nonstick skillet. Cook for 15 minutes on each side. Store the leftovers in the freezer and warm in microwave when needed.

Eggplant Roll-Ups

A dish you can enjoy without the guilt of too many carbohydrates or too much fat. This dish is great for diabetics or for anyone who wants to lose weight.

    2 large eggplants
    salt
    16-ounce package of firm tofu
    32-ounce spaghetti sauce
    1 tablespoon garlic powder
    1 tablespoon onion powder
    1 tablespoon rosemary
    2 tablespoons Braggs amino or soy sauce

Cut off both ends of the eggplants and then longitudinally slice, 1/4 of an inch thick. Place slices on oiled baking sheet and then sprinkle salt to taste. Allow to bake for about 15 minutes on each side. In a large mixing bowl, place tofu, mashed or scrambled with a fork. Add powdered spices and rosemary and then mix well. Add Braggs amino or soy sauce and mix (taste and add salt if needed). Place a full tablespoon of tofu on one end of each side of eggplant and roll. Add a thin layer of spaghetti sauce at the bottom of the baking dish, and cover with the remaining spaghetti sauce. Cover with foil and bake for 45 minutes.

Eggplant Zucchini Bake

Delicious and packed with vitamins and fiber, this dish is great for everyone, but is especially ideal for diabetic or those who are trying to lose weight.

    2 tablespoons olive oil
    4 large zucchini (1-inch cubes)

    2 medium eggplants (1-inch cubes)
    2 cups cherry tomatoes (cut in halves)
    1 small onion, chopped
    1 tablespoon garlic powder
    1/4 cup basil, fresh
    1/4 cup parsley
    salt to taste

Place oil in casserole dish and add zucchini, eggplant, and cherry tomatoes. Add other ingredients. Salt to taste and mix. Bake for 30 minutes, uncovered. Then cover with foil and bake for another 15 minutes.

Cauliflower White Bean Mashed

This is a great dish for diabetics. It has complex carbohydrates, fiber, protein, and good fat.

    8 cups cauliflower florets, fresh or frozen
    1 (15-ounce) can white or lima beans
    2/3 cup of cashew, raw (optional)
    2 teaspoons onion powder
    2 teaspoons garlic powder

In a medium-sized pot, cook cauliflower for about 6 minutes. Pat dry with paper towel. Do not allow the cauliflower to become cold. Warm the beans on medium heat. Then place in food processor with the cashews. Process for a few minutes, then add cauliflower and continue to process until smooth.

Five-Grain Brown Rice Pilaf

This is a complete dish, filled with complex carbohydrates, protein, and fiber.

1 medium onion, chopped

3 cloves garlic, mashed and diced

4 1/2 cups vegetable broth or water, warmed

1 1/2 cups long-grain brown rice

1/2 cup lentils

1/2 cup quinoa

1/4 cup bulbar wheat

1/4 cup couscous

1 tablespoon McKay's chicken-style seasoning

salt, to taste

Sauté in rice cooker or saucepan, half a cup of vegetable broth, onion, and garlic for 2 to 3 minutes. Stir in slowly the rice and grains for 2 minutes. Then add water or vegetable broth, salt, and McKay's seasoning and bring to a boil. Reduce heat, cover, and allow to simmer for 45 to 55 minutes. Remove from heat and allow to stand for another 10 minutes. This mixture could also be poured into a casserole dish, covered, and baked at 350 degrees Fahrenheit for 50 to 60 minutes.

Seasoned Vegetable Rice

This colorful dish goes well with beans or no-meat meatballs.

4 cups brown basmati rice, cooked

1 teaspoon extra-virgin olive oil

1 clove garlic, minced

1 small onion, chopped

2 to 3 teaspoons McKay's chicken-style seasoning

2 cups broccoli, finely chopped

2 cups carrots, shredded

1/4 cup vegetable broth

salt, to taste

Cook the basmati rice according to the package directions. In a pot, over medium heat, sauté for 2 to 3 minutes garlic and onions in oil. Add vegetables and McKay's seasoning, then simmer for about 5 to 7 minutes. Additional vegetable broth may be added if needed. Add the cooked basmati rice and simmer for 7 to 10 minutes. Taste the mixture and add salt to taste. Serve with any protein dish of your choice.

Wild Rice and Mushroom Pilaf

Wild rice has a low glycemic index; therefore, this dish will not significantly raise the blood sugar.

> 1/2 cup green onions, finely chopped
> 1/2 cup celery, chopped
> 3 cups sliced mushrooms
> 1 cup wild rice
> 1 1/2 teaspoons McKay's chicken-style seasoning
> 3 cups pure water or broth
> 1 cup sliced almonds, slightly toasted

In a medium-sized covered pan, sauté the onions and celery in a little olive oil until tender. Stir in mushrooms, wild rice, almonds, and seasoning; sauté for 2 to 3 minutes. Carefully add the water or broth, and bring to a boil. Reduce heat, cover, and simmer for about 50 minutes until rice is tender and liquid is absorbed. Leave covered for 10 minutes. Fluff with a fork before serving and garnish with more almonds, if desired.

Indian Rice

Add fresh vegetables to this delicious rice dish and enjoy.

> 1 medium onion, chopped
> 2 cloves garlic, mashed and diced

1/2 cup carrots, chopped

1/4 cup slivered almonds

2 1/2 cups boiling water

1 cup long-grain brown rice

1/2 cup frozen green beans

1/2 cup frozen corn

1 teaspoon cumin

1/4 tablespoon ginger powder

2 teaspoons turmeric

1 tablespoon McKay's chicken-style seasoning

salt, to taste

Preheat the oven to 350 degrees Fahrenheit. Sauté the onion, garlic, and carrots for about 5 minutes. Add the rice and other ingredients, stirring together gently. Add the boiling water and pour into a 1 1/2-quart casserole dish. Bake, covered, for 50 to 55 minutes. Lightly toast the almonds in a dry, nonstick skillet, and then stir them in with rice mixture. Serve with a bean salad or chickpea curry.

Seasoned Black Bean Brown Rice

If you enjoy black beans, then this is a great dish for you.

1 medium onion, chopped

3 cloves garlic, mashed and diced

2 cups long-grain uncooked brown rice

1 (15-ounce) can black beans

4 cups water

2 teaspoons thyme

1 tablespoon McKay's chicken-style seasoning

1 tablespoon Mrs. Dash, salt-free seasoning

Preheat oven to 350 degrees Fahrenheit. On low heat, sauté for 2 to 3 minutes the onion and garlic in a small amount of water. Add in the rice, black beans, and other ingredients. Continue to sauté for another 3 minutes. Now add the 4 cups of water. Pour mixture in a casserole dish, cover, and place in preheated oven at 350 degrees Fahrenheit for 60 minutes. Use as a main dish or serve with a fresh vegetable salad.

Chickpea Avocado Spread

This spread make a wholesome and delicious sandwich. Just add tomato, spinach leaves, and alfalfa sprouts.

> 1 medium avocado
> 15 ounce chickpeas
> 1 tablespoon lemon juice
> 1/2 sweet onion
> salt to taste

Remove peel and seed from avocado. Drain and rinse chickpeas. Add all the ingredients to the food processor and process until smooth. Can be used as sandwich spread or dip.

Lentil Walnut Meatballs

These look and taste better than meat. Cook in tomato sauce and serve over whole wheat spaghetti.

> 1 cup soaked lentils (cover in water and soak overnight)
> 1/4 cup walnuts, chopped
> 1/2 cup onion, chopped
> 1 teaspoon thyme
> 1 teaspoon cumin
> 2 tablespoons tahini

1 teaspoon garlic powder

1/2 cup oat flour

1 teaspoon sage

1 teaspoon salt

1 teaspoon fresh basil, finely chopped

Pour off the water and then blend lentil to a paste. Place lentils in a bowl. Add all the other ingredients and mix together. Form small balls and then place them on a baking tray. Preheat oven to 200 degrees Fahrenheit, and bake for approximately 20 to 25 minutes.

Meatball Tomato Sauce

1 1/2 cups tomato puree

1/2 cup onion, chopped

1 clove garlic, mashed and diced

2 teaspoons sweet paprika

1 1/2 teaspoons thyme, dried

1 1/2 cups water

2 tablespoons fresh basil, chopped

salt to taste

Place 2 tablespoons of water in nonstick pan on low-medium heat. Add onion and garlic. Sauté for 2 to 3 minutes and add the other ingredients. Continue to sauté for another 3 minutes. Then add meatballs. Enjoy with whole-grain spaghetti.

Pasta Primavera

Another great source of vitamins and phytochemicals. This dish will empower you as you seek to keep diseases in retreat! Be careful not to overcook your veggies. Too much heat will destroy some of the nutrients in these foods.

> 1 tablespoon olive oil
> 1/2 cup onion, thinly sliced
> 2 cloves garlic, mashed and then minced
> 1/2 cup red or yellow bell pepper, sliced
> 1/2 cup carrots, julienned
> 2 cups cauliflower florets
> 1 bunch broccoli florets
> 1 medium zucchini, sliced
> 1 teaspoon salt or to taste
> 1 cup tomatoes, diced
> 1 box (16 ounces) pasta, cooked, using instructions on package
> 1 recipe Alfredo sauce
> 1/4 cup nondairy parmesan cheese or nutritional yeast flakes (optional)

In a large saucepan, heat oil over medium heat. Add onion, garlic, carrots, and bell pepper. Cook until softened (about 4 minutes). Add cauliflower, broccoli, zucchini, and salt. Stir occasionally. Cook until vegetables are ready (about 5 minutes).

Prepare pasta using instructions from the package. Add pasta and sauce to the vegetables. Gently mix together and cook until heated through. Top with tomatoes and nondairy parmesan cheese.

Pasta with Vegetables

Be creative and use the vegetables that you enjoy. Using vegetables of many colors will give different vitamins, minerals, and phytonutrients, which are all essential for disease prevention or reversal.

> 2 tablespoons olive oil

1/2 cup red onion, diced

2 cloves garlic, mashed and minced

4 stalks celery, diced

1 cup carrots, julienned

1 pound fresh asparagus or green beans, cut in 1-inch pieces

1 medium zucchini, thinly sliced

1 cup leafy greens

3 tablespoons Braggs amino or soy sauce

2 cups vegetable broth

1/2 tablespoon cornstarch

1 package (14 ounces) whole-grain angel hair pasta, cooked using directions on package

2 cups tomatoes, chopped

6 to 8 leaves fresh basil or 1 teaspoon dried basil

1/2 teaspoon dried oregano

Heat oil in wok over medium heat. Add onion, garlic, celery, and carrots. Cook until softened, stirring occasionally, about 7 to 8 minutes. Add asparagus, zucchini, and salt. Cook until vegetables are just softened, about 4 minutes. Whisk cornstarch and broth together in a small bowl. Add broth and remaining ingredients to wok. Bring to a boil over high heat and cook until thickened.

Veggie Wrap with Guacamole

Here is another menu in which you want to use your creativity. Choose veggies that you enjoy. Prepare veggies ahead, and then the rest is easy. This is a complete meal with vegetables, protein, carbohydrates, and good fat.

finely grate any vegetables

carrots

cabbage

butternut squash

slice any of the following
sweet peppers
onions
mushrooms
sprouts of your choice
nuts of your choice

one batch of tahini sauce
one batch of guacamole

Bake wrap for 15 seconds in a very hot pan (without oil) to prevent from breaking when rolling. Spread guacamole in a rectangle in the middle of the tortilla. Put your choice of vegetable on the guacamole, and fold like an envelope, leaving the top side open. Put some tahini sauce on, close your envelope, and enjoy.

Chickpea Curry

This is another recipe the patients at my Wellness Center enjoy. It goes well with steamed brown rice. It is somewhat spicy, so feel free to decrease the amount of ginger or cayenne pepper that the recipe calls for.

2 tablespoons olive oil
1 onion, chopped
2 cloves garlic, mashed then minced
2 teaspoons fresh ginger root, finely chopped
2 teaspoons cumin
1 teaspoon ground coriander
1 teaspoon sage
sea salt to taste
1 teaspoon cayenne pepper

1 tablespoon ground turmeric

2 (15-ounce) cans chickpeas

1/2 cup water

Heat oil in a large saucepan over medium heat. Add onion and spices. Sauté until tender. Then add beans and water. Cook for 20 minutes.

Lentil Patties

These are absolutely delicious. You will not miss the meat. Serve on a bun or with gravy over rice or baked potato or with mixed vegetables.

2 cups cooked red lentils, drained

1/2 cup onions, finely chopped

1 teaspoon dried thyme

1 cup finely ground chia seeds

1/4 cup brown rice flour or oatmeal flour

2 teaspoons sea salt

1 teaspoon garlic powder

1 teaspoon onion powder

1 1/4 teaspoon sage

1 cup grated carrots

1 cup pecans

175 grams tiny mushrooms, drained and chopped

1 cup water or milk

1 cup celery, finely chopped

Line your baking pan with parchment paper or spray your pan with oil. Mix all the ingredients together and make patties. Put patties on the baking pan. Bake at 350 degrees Fahrenheit for 30 minutes. Turn them over after 20 minutes. Hint—use an ice cream scoop and make balls instead of patties and bake.

Walnut Balls

This recipe makes 24 balls.

> 4 cups water
> 4 cups rolled oats
> 1 medium onion, finely chopped
> 4 garlic cloves
> 1/2 cup raw sunflower seeds
> 1/2 cup Braggs aminos
> 1/2 cup walnuts, chopped
> 1/4 cup olive oil
> 1 tablespoon molasses
> 1/2 cup nutritional yeast
> 1 tablespoon Italian seasoning
> 1 teaspoon ground coriander
> 1 teaspoon dried sage

Boil 4 cups of water. Mix the hot water with all the other ingredients and let sit in the bowl for 10 minutes. Shape into balls. Put in the baking dish and bake at 350 degrees Fahrenheit for 20 to 30 minutes. These walnut balls taste better the next day. Freeze well.

Chinese Stir-Fry Vegetables

This dish is very colorful with many different vegetables. This indicates that you will receive various nutrients from this one dish. Serve with brown rice.

> olive-oil spray
> 1 pound (16 ounces) tofu, firm, cut into bite-sized cubes
> 1 medium to large onion, sliced
> 2/3 cup carrots, julienned

1 cup cauliflower florets

1/4 cup water

2/3 cup celery, cut in 3-inch pieces

1 cup broccoli florets

1/2 cup bean sprouts

2/3 cup snow pea pods

1 can water chestnuts

1 can baby corn cobs

2/3 cup bok choy, chopped

2 tablespoons chicken-like seasoning of your choice, to taste

2 tablespoons Braggs amino or soy sauce

Spray small amount of oil in wok or nonstick skillet and then place it on medium-high heat. When oil is hot, add tofu. Slightly braze tofu, allowing each piece to become slightly brown. Then remove and place aside. Now add onion to wok or skillet and sauté for 2 minutes. Then add vegetables. First add the carrots and the cauliflower and allow to cook for 3 to 5 minutes. May need to add a small amount of water. Now add the other vegetables. Stir intermittently, allowing all the vegetables to be cooked evenly for 3 minutes. Add tofu, chicken-style seasoning, and Braggs amino or soy sauce. Continue to stir and allow to cook for 2 minutes more. Take care not to overcook the vegetables.

Sun-Dried Tomatoes, Black Beans, and Rice Salad

This very delicious dish is packed with protein, fiber, complex carbohydrates, and good fat. Goes well with raw vegetables and is great to prevent diabetes, heart disease, and obesity.

2 1/2 cups long-grained brown rice, cooked

1/2 cup marinated sun-dried tomatoes, coarsely chopped

1 ripe avocado, diced

1/2 cup black beans, cooked

    1 stalk celery, finely chopped
    1/4 cup almond slivers
    3 leaves fresh basil, julienned
    1 tablespoon fresh lemon juice
    1 tablespoon garlic powder
    1 tablespoon diced red onion
    1 teaspoon salt

In a large mixing bowl, combine all ingredients and mix well.

Mock Tuna Salad

This is a great dish for a party or any social event. It is delicious and easy to prepare. It may be served on whole wheat bread with lettuce. Leftovers can be stored in the refrigerator for 3 to 4 days.

    1 (15-ounce) can of chickpeas, drained
    1/4 cup reduced-fat vegenaise
    1/3 cup celery, finely chopped
    2 tablespoons sweet onion, finely chopped
    1/2 tablespoon nutritional yeast flakes
    1 teaspoon low-sodium soy sauce

In a medium bowl, mash the chickpeas with a fork and combine with the rest of the ingredients.

Black Bean, Corn, and Quinoa Salad

Quinoa is a whole grain that has a high-protein and high-fiber content. It is great for those seeking to stay healthy for life.

    1 tablespoon extra-virgin olive oil
    1 onion, chopped

3 cloves garlic, minced

1/4 cup quinoa, uncooked

1 1/2 cups vegetable broth (low sodium)

1 tablespoon ground cumin

1/4 tablespoon cayenne pepper

salt to taste

2 cups frozen corn kernels

2 (15-ounce) cans black beans, rinsed and drained

1/2 cup fresh cilantro, chopped

2 tablespoons lime or lemon juice

1 jalapeno, seeded and diced finely (optional)

Over the medium heat, heat oil in a saucepan and sauté the onion and garlic until they're soft and translucent. Add the quinoa to the pan and cover with vegetable broth. Season with cumin, cayenne pepper, and salt. Then bring the mixture to a boil. Cover, reduce the heat, and simmer for 20 minutes, stirring occasionally. Add the frozen corn to the pan and continue to simmer for 5 more minutes. Mix in the black beans, cilantro, lime juice, and optional jalapeno and cook until beans are heated through.

Quinoa Salad

This is a salad that everyone enjoys. It is packed with minerals, vitamins, healthy fat, and complex carbohydrates. All these nutrients will help to keep diseases in retreat.

2 cups quinoa

4 cups water

1 green bell pepper, chopped

1/4 cup chopped red onion

1/2 cup seedless grapes in halves

1 cup cherry tomatoes in halves

1 medium cucumber (cubed)

1/4 cup walnuts (optional)
1/4 cup fresh mint (chopped)

Rinse the quinoa well before cooking. Place the quinoa and water in a saucepan. Bring to a boil, cover, and reduce the heat. Simmer for about 15 minutes or until the liquid is absorbed. Then allow quinoa to cool. Combine the chopped vegetables in a bowl, including the fresh chopped herb of your choice. Mix well. Add the cooked quinoa. Toss gently and add dressing of your choice. Toss again and add pepper to taste. Cover and chill for at least 2 hours before serving.

Spicy Mexican Beans

May use as filling for tacos, burritos, or enchiladas or served as a side dish.

1 onion, finely chopped
2 cloves garlic
2 (15-ounce) cans pintos beans
1 teaspoon cumin
2 teaspoons chili powder
1 teaspoon cayenne powder
3 tablespoons water

Place saucepan on medium heat. Sauté the onion and garlic in 2 tablespoons water for 3 minutes. Lower heat and then add the other ingredients and stir. Allow to cook for about 8 to 10 minutes. Remove from heat and allow to form a few minutes. Place beans in a food processor and pulse a few times until desired consistency is achieved.

Corn and Potato Chowder

3 cups water
3 cups potatoes

1/3 cup carrots, diced

1 cup green onion, chopped

1 1/2 teaspoons sea salt

1 1/2 teaspoons rosemary

1 teaspoon all-purpose or McKay's chicken-style seasoning

3 cups creamed or liquefied fresh corn

1 tablespoon nut butter, blended with corn

3/4 cup green pepper, chopped

In a soup pot, bring all ingredients except corn to a boil. Reduce heat and simmer to almost tender. Add blended corn and nut butter. Simmer for 8 to 10 minutes more. Garnish with fresh minced parsley, chives, or dill weed. Serve with soup crackers or breadsticks.

Soups

Quinoa Lentil Soup

This recipe is simply delicious and healthy. It is packed with fiber, protein, vitamins, and minerals. Just an ideal dish for disease reversal!

    1 cup quinoa
    2 cups lentils, cooked
    10 cups water
    2 cups corn
    3 cups cabbage, chopped in large pieces
    2 cups carrots, thinly sliced
    3 cloves garlic, mashed and then minced
    2 cups onions, chopped
    5 tablespoons chicken-like seasoning
    1 teaspoon Mrs. Dash seasoning

Place all ingredients in a large pot and cook for about 30 minutes or until carrots are cooked. Serve hot.

Thai Coconut Curry Soup

    1 large onion, chopped
    1 clove garlic, mashed and minced
    1 red or orange bell pepper, chopped
    1/4 head cauliflower, chopped
    2 red potatoes, diced
    1/3 head cabbage, chopped
    1 cup green beans, diced
    1 cup carrots, cubed
    2 cans coconut milk
    4 cups water or vegetable broth

2 tablespoons curry powder

1 teaspoon turmeric

1 tablespoon olive oil

2 tablespoons McKay's chicken-style seasoning or other savory seasoning

1/2 teaspoon salt

1 tablespoon fresh grated ginger

1/2 teaspoon turmeric

Place oil in a large pot on medium heat, sauté onion and garlic for 2 minutes. Then add all vegetables. Add the coconut milk and water or vegetable broth, and bring to a boil. Now incorporate the remaining ingredients, reduce heat, cover pot, and allow to cook until vegetables are tender. Taste and add salt, if desired. May garnish with chopped green onion.

Creamy Potato Broccoli Soup

2 cups onion, chopped

7 cups of water

2 1/2 pounds potatoes, peeled and diced

3 cups broccoli florets, cooked

1 cup raw cashews

2 tablespoons McKay's chicken-style seasonings

2 teaspoons garlic powder

1 teaspoon salt or to taste

1 tablespoon fresh thyme, chopped

In a large pot, sauté onion in small amount of water. Then add six cups of water, add potatoes, cover, and allow to cook on medium to high for 15 minutes. Remove outer skin from broccoli stems and add broccoli to soup. Blend cashew nuts in 1 cup of water until smooth. When potatoes are cooked, add cashew mixture to pot. Also, add all the spices and other ingredients. Stir occasionally and allow to cook for another 5 minutes.

Remove 1/2 the soup (potatoes and broccoli) and blend. Then return this blended mixture to pot. Serve hot.

Kale and White Bean Soup

Soups are usually filling and supply only a few calories. This dish is packed with protein, fiber, vitamins, minerals, and antioxidants.

olive oil spray
1 medium onion, diced
4 cloves garlic, minced
4 cups vegetable broth (low sodium)
4 cups kale, ribs removed, chopped
2 large carrots, sliced in 1/4-inch coins
1 (15-ounce) can Italian-style diced tomatoes
1 teaspoon, fresh thyme, chopped
2 (15-ounce) cans white beans, drained and rinsed
1 teaspoon Italian seasoning
salt, to taste

In a large pot, cook the onions with olive oil over medium heat for about 3 minutes. Add the garlic and cook for 2 minutes more. When the onion and garlic are translucent, add the vegetable broth, kale, tomatoes, carrots, Italian seasoning and thyme. Then cover. Cook until carrots and kale are tender, about 15 to 20 minutes. Add the white beans, salt to taste, and cook until beans are heated through. Serve hot.

Italian White Bean Soup

This is another great recipe. Feel free to incorporate the vegetables and spices that you enjoy. Serve hot.

1 teaspoon extra-virgin olive oil

2 cloves garlic, minced

1 cup water

1 (32-ounce) can great northern beans, liquid reserved

1 to 2 teaspoons McKay's chicken-style instant broth and seasoning

3/4 cup of celery, chopped

3/4 cup of carrots, chopped

1 teaspoon fresh thyme, chopped

In a medium pot, sauté the garlic in olive oil for 2 to 3 minutes. When the garlic is cooked, add the remaining ingredients and simmer for 10 minutes more.

Zucchini and Cauliflower Soup

This is a great dish that has vegetables, which are low in calories, so enjoy and keep the weight off. This dish is also great for those who want to keep the blood sugar down. These vegetables have very low glycemic index values.

6 medium zucchini, chopped

5 cups water / vegetable broth

1 small onion, chopped

2 cloves garlic, mashed and minced

2 tablespoons savory seasoning

1/2 cup soy milk or 1/4 cup soymilk powder

1 teaspoon fresh thyme, chopped

3 cups cauliflower florets, chopped

Place the zucchini, cauliflower, water, onion, garlic, and thyme in a saucepan and cook over medium heat until the vegetables are tender, about 15 minutes. Add the remaining ingredients. Blend the soup in batches in a blender or food processor until smooth. Serve at once, or reheat just before serving.

Split Pea Soup

This is one of my favorite soup recipes. It is high in fiber and protein content.

2 cups split peas
4–5 cups water
2 tablespoons pearl barley
2 carrots, sliced or diced
2 celery stalks, diced
1 onion, chopped
1/2 teaspoon sea salt or to taste
2 cloves garlic, mashed then minced
3 sprigs fresh thyme
1/2 teaspoon Mrs. Dash
1 teaspoon savory seasoning of your choice
2 to 3 bay leaves

Cover the split peas with 4 to 5 cups of water and allow to cook for 15 minutes on medium heat. Add the rest of the ingredients. Simmer until tender and creamy, stirring often. Last, add 1/2 tablespoon olive oil (optional). Taste and add extra spice if needed. Serve hot.

Italian Minestrone

Vegetable soup is a great way to consume the recommended daily servings (5 to 6) of vegetables in one meal.

10 cups pure water, boiling
1 large onion, sliced
4 medium carrots, sliced
2 cups cabbage or fennel, chopped
2 large celery stalks, sliced or diced

1 (10 ounce) package frozen cut green beans

1/2 cup elbow noodles

1 (15-ounce) can kidney beans

3 garlic cloves, mashed and minced

1 (10-ounce) package frozen peas

1 (15-ounce) can kidney beans or chickpeas

1 (28-ounce) can Italian tomatoes, cut

1 bay leaf

4 sprigs of parsley

4 sprigs of sweet basil

2 teaspoons of salt

Bring water to boil. Add all ingredients except noodles. Simmer for 30 minutes, and then add noodles. Continue to simmer for 15 minutes, stirring occasionally until noodles are tender. May sprinkle vegan parmesan cheese before serving, if desired.

Lentil Soup with Vegetables

This is a great dish to serve on a cold winter day. You can add other vegetables if desired. Serve with whole wheat bread.

2 cups lentils

1 1/2 cups onion, chopped

2 cup carrots, cubed

2 large potatoes, cubed

8 cups water

1/2 cup celery, chopped

2 tablespoons savory seasoning

4 garlic cloves, minced

1 bay leaf

2 teaspoon Italian herbs or Mrs. Dash

1 teaspoon thyme

In a large pot, combine the lentils and water and allow to cook for about 60 minutes until lentils are tender. Then add the vegetables and all the other ingredients. Allow to cook for another 30 minutes, stirring occasionally. Serve hot.

Indian Lentil Soup

1 cup dry red lentils
5 cups of water
1 garlic clove, crushed
1 tablespoon olive oil
1 cup onion, chopped
1/2 cup celery, thinly sliced
1 cup carrots, finely diced
15-ounce can chunky tomatoes
1 bay leaf
1/8 teaspoon chili powder
1 1/2 teaspoons salt
1/2 cup fresh parsley, chopped

Combine lentils, water, garlic, oil, onion, celery, and carrots in a soup pot and bring to a boil. Reduce heat; cover and let simmer for 1 hour. Add the tomatoes, bay leaf, chili powder, and salt and let simmer a few more minutes. Just before serving, remove the bay leaf and add parsley.

Quinoa Lentil Soup

This soup is simply delicious and is complete with complex carbohydrates, protein, fiber, vitamins and minerals.

2 cups carrots, thinly sliced
1 cup quinoa

2 cups lentils, cooked

10 cups of water

2 cups frozen corn

3 cups cabbage, chopped

3 garlic cloves, mashed and minced

2 cups onion, chopped

5 tablespoons chicken-like seasoning, such as McKay's chicken-style seasoning

1 teaspoon Mrs. Dash

In a large pot, cook the carrots for about 12 minutes and then add the other ingredients and continue cooking for another 20 minutes. Serve hot.

Jamaican Kidney Bean Soup

This dish is commonly served in the typical Jamaican home or restaurant. The elbow noodles are used to replace spinners. You can add a small slice of scotch bonnet pepper to give it the authentic Jamaican flavor.

10 cups of water (better to use water from the cooked beans)

2 cups carrots, sliced

2 cups potatoes, cubed

1 cup coconut milk

3 cups red kidney beans, freshly cooked

3 garlic cloves, mashed and minced

1 cup onion, chopped

4 green onions, chopped

1 teaspoon Mrs. Dash seasoning

5 tablespoons McKay's chicken-style seasoning

4–6 sprigs fresh thyme

1 cup whole wheat elbow noodles

In a large pot, place water, carrots, potatoes, and coconut milk and allow to cook for 30 minutes. Then add all the other ingredients and allow to cook an additional 20 minutes on low to medium heat.

Spinach Kale Soup

This dish is tasty, packed with antioxidants, and very filling. Serve hot.

> 1/2 pound yellow yam or 2 large potatoes or yucca
> 12 okras, cut in 1-inch cubes
> 8–10 cups water or vegetable stock
> 2 (10-ounce) packages spinach, frozen
> 2 cups kale, chopped
> 2 garlic cloves, mashed and minced
> 1/2 cup coconut milk
> 2 green onions, chopped
> 1 teaspoon Mrs. Dash seasoning
> 2 tablespoons beef-like seasoning
> 2 tablespoons Braggs amino or soy sauce
> 4 sprigs of fresh thyme
> salt to taste

Peel yellow yam, yucca, or potato and cut in 1-inch cubes and set aside. Wash okras, cut in 1-inch cubes, and set aside. In a large pot, add the water or vegetable stock and then add spinach and kale. Cook for 10 to 15 minutes. Take out the spinach and kale and blend in a food processor or blender and then set aside. Now add the okras, yam, potato, or yucca and garlic to stock and allow to cook on medium heat for 30 minutes. Now add the spinach-kale mixture, with green onion, thyme, coconut milk, and spices and allow to simmer for 15 minutes. Serve hot.

Cream of Pumpkin Soup

1 tablespoon olive oil
1 medium onion, chopped
2 cups soy milk
3 tablespoons whole-grain flour
1 teaspoon Mrs. Dash
2 cups (1 pound) boiled pureed pumpkin
salt to taste

On low heat sauté in hot oil the onion for 2 minutes. Then add flour and Mrs. Dash. Add milk slowly and continue to stir until smooth and thickened. Combine pumpkin with mixture. Simmer for 5 minutes. Serve hot.

Lentil Stew

This is a very simple but tasty dish. Serve over cooked brown rice, quinoa, or couscous or with potato, accompanied by a green salad.

2 cups uncooked lentil
6 cups water
1 large onion, chopped
4 cloves garlic mashed and diced
2 tablespoons thyme, fresh or dry
2 teaspoons Mrs. Dash (salt free)
2 teaspoons McKay's seasoning
2 tablespoons vegetable oil (optional)

Place lentils in large, deep pot. Add 6 cups water. Cook on medium heat for 90 minutes. Then add all the other ingredients. Allow to cook for another 30 minutes.

Easy Green Pea Soup

This soup is absolutely simple and easy to prepare. Serve as side dish for lunch or dinner.

    1/3 cup cashews or walnuts, raw
    3 cups vegetable stock or water
    1 (15-ounce) can peas (bean)
    1/2 medium onion
    1 tablespoon flour
    salt to taste

Blend nuts in vegetable stock until smooth. Then add other ingredients continue to blend until smooth. Heat mixture just enough until flour is cooked. Then serve hot.

Summer Soup

Here is a cold soup you may relish on a hot summer day or evening. It is absolutely delicious and ideal for those who want to maintain a healthy weight and normal blood sugar.

    2 cups water
    1 pound tomatoes, ripe
    1/2 medium cucumber
    1/4 medium onion
    2 stalks celery
    1/2 teaspoon salt
    1/8 cup cashews, raw
    pinch of cayenne pepper

Wash vegetables and then blend all ingredients and water in a high-speed blender. Chill in refrigerator before serving. Serves 4.

Cream of Broccoli Soup

2 scallion (green onions) stalks, washed and sliced
2 cloves garlic, minced
1 1/2 cup vegetable stock
4 medium red potatoes, peeled and chopped
2 cups almond milk
2 medium stalks of broccoli, one chopped and one cut into small florets
1/2 teaspoon fresh thyme
1 teaspoon oregano
freshly ground pepper to taste
pinch of nutmeg

Sauté the leek and garlic in 1/3 cup of stock for 5 minutes. Add the remaining ingredients except the broccoli florets. Cover and cook over medium heat for 40 minutes or until potatoes are tender. Blend the mixture, in batches, in a blender or food processor until smooth and creamy. Return to the pan and keep warm. Meanwhile, place the broccoli florets in another saucepan with water to cover. Cover and cook over medium heat for 5 minutes. Drain. Add to the soup mixture. Season with freshly ground pepper to taste.

Sauces, Gravies, and Dips

Cashew Cheese Sauce

This delicious cheese sauce is cholesterol free and is full of good healthy fats. This can be used as a spread or for macaroni and cheese. It is also great with steamed broccoli.

    2 cups water
    1/2 cup clean, raw cashews
    2-ounce jar pimientos, sliced or diced
    3 tablespoons food yeast flakes
    2 tablespoons cornstarch
    2 tablespoons fresh lemon juice
    1 1/2 teaspoon salt
    1 teaspoon onion flakes or powder
    1 teaspoon garlic powder

Blend cashews in about 1/2 cup of water until very smooth. Add remaining water and other ingredients and continue blending until smooth. Simmer in a heavy saucepan until thickened, stirring constantly (5 to 6 min). Yields 2 1/2 cups or 10 servings.

Alfredo Sauce

This is a great nondairy option. Feel free to add other herbs that you like.

    1/2 cup cashew nuts
    1 3/4 cups water
    1 tablespoon of cornstarch
    1 teaspoon garlic powder
    1 teaspoon onion powder
    1 tablespoon chicken-like seasoning

1/2 teaspoon oregano

Place all ingredients into a blender. Blend until smooth. Place in a medium-sized pot. Simmer on low heat, and stir continuously until thickened and smooth. Add salt to taste. Pour over pasta or enjoy with baked potato.

Lima Bean Cheese Sauce

This is a great cheese sauce for those who might have a nut allergy. It has a good amount of fiber and protein.

    15 ounces lima beans (cooked)
    3/4 cup nutritional yeast flakes
    3/4 cup soy milk (plain)
    2 teaspoons onion powder
    2 teaspoons of garlic powder
    1/2 teaspoon paprika
    1/2 teaspoon turmeric
    1 teaspoon salt (or to taste)
    1 small onion (chopped)
    1 medium red bell pepper
    1 tablespoon vegetable oil

Place all the ingredients except the onion and bell pepper in blender and blend until smooth. Sauté onion and bell pepper in oil on low heat for 2 to 3 minutes. Then add to pot and simmer on low heat for 7 to 10 minutes.

Tofu Cheese Sauce

This sauce can be used as a dip for raw vegetables but is also excellent for macaroni and cheese.

    1/2 cup of raw cashew

1 pack firm tofu

3/4 cup nutritional yeast flakes

3 cups of water

1 large red bell pepper

2 tablespoons Bragg amino sauce

1 teaspoon turmeric

2 cloves garlic (mashed)

1 large onion (chopped)

1 tablespoon savory seasoning

1 1/2 teaspoons salt

2 tablespoons cornstarch

Blend cashew nuts with water. Then add the remaining ingredients and blend until smooth. Simmer on low heat for 7 to 10 minutes. Stir continuously until thickened.

Cheese Sauce

This sauce can be served over pasta or poured over broccoli.

3/4 cup diced cooked carrots

3/4 cup diced cooked potatoes

1/2 cup nutritional yeast flakes

1/2 teaspoon paprika

1 teaspoon garlic powder

2 teaspoons onion powder

1 cup water

1 small onion (cooked)

1 teaspoon salt

Blend all ingredients until smooth.

Mango Avocado Salsa

Delicious salsa, best served with healthy tortilla chips or as a side dish for Mexican cuisine.

    1 mango, peeled, seeded, and diced
    1 avocado, peeled, pitted, and diced
    4 medium tomatoes, diced
    1 jalapeño pepper, seeded and diced
    1/2 cup chopped fresh cilantro
    3 cloves garlic, minced
    1 teaspoon salt
    2 tablespoons fresh lime juice
    1/4 cup chopped red onion

In a medium bowl, combine the mango, avocado, tomatoes, jalapeño, cilantro, and garlic. Stir in the salt, lime juice, and red onion. Allow to stand in refrigerator for 30 minutes before serving.

Guacamole

Please watch your portion size. Avocado has good fats, but this dish is high in calories.

    1 avocado, large
    2 tablespoons lemon juice
    2 tablespoons onion (chopped)
    1/2 teaspoon salt

Remove the skin and pit, cut avocado into small pieces, and mash with a fork. Add the remaining ingredients and mix well. Guacamole tends to become brown when exposed to air. To prevent this, store with the pit. Serve with Mexican dishes like tacos, nachos, burritos, or rice and beans.

Chickpea Spread or Dip

This is better made the day before you plan to serve it and refrigerated. Use as a sandwich spread or as a dip for pita bread.

    1/4 cup water
    1–3 teaspoons ground cumin (to taste)
    2 tablespoons lemon juice
    1–2 garlic cloves
    water-packed chickpeas, drained and rinsed
    1 small sweet onion
    chili powder to taste (optional)

Combine the ingredients in a blender and process until smooth.

Mushroom Gravy

Great low-fat gravy that can be served over meatballs.

    1/2 cup onions (chopped)
    2 cloves garlic, mashed then minced
    2 cups mushrooms, fresh (sliced)
    4 cups soy milk
    1 tablespoon Braggs amino or soy sauce
    3 tablespoons whole wheat flour
    1 teaspoon basil or sage

Sauté garlic, onions, and mushrooms in a medium pot, using a small amount of water. Then add the remaining ingredients. Whisk flour in slowly to prevent clumping. Simmer for another 5 to 7 minutes until thickened.

Almond Nut Gravy

This ultra-low-fat gravy is very easy to prepare. Save leftover in the refrigerator.

  1/2 cup almonds
  2 cups water
  2 tablespoons McKay's chicken-style seasoning
  2 tablespoons Braggs amino soy
  1 tablespoon nutritional yeast
  1/2 teaspoon garlic powder
  1/2 teaspoon onion powder
  2 tablespoons cornstarch
  1 small onion
  1/2 teaspoon dry basil

Place all ingredients in a high-speed blender with 1 3/4 cup of water. Blend until smooth. Place mixture in a saucepan and allow to simmer on medium heat. Mix cornstarch in remaining water and incorporate to mixture. Stir frequently until smooth. Serve with lentil patties or loaf or baked potatoes.

Country-Style Brown Gravy

This gravy is simple and easy to make. You can enjoy it over lentil patties, meatloaf, or meatballs.

  2 cups warm water
  3 cloves garlic, mashed then minced
  1/8 cup cashew pieces, rinsed
  1/2 teaspoon garlic powder
  1 tablespoon onion powder
  1/2 teaspoon Italian herbs
  2 tablespoons cornstarch

  3 sprigs fresh thyme
  1/2 tomato, chopped
  3 tablespoons soy sauce
  1 tablespoon parsley

Place 1/2 cup warm water and all the ingredients except the parsley in a blender or food processor and blend until smooth and creamy. When creamy, add 1 1/2 cups more warm water and blend. Pour into a saucepan and cook over low-medium heat, stirring constantly, until thick (about 5 minutes).

SALAD DRESSINGS

Cucumber Salad Dressing

Easy to make, this delicious dressing goes well on green vegetables.

  3 small cucumbers
  2 tablespoons fresh lemon juice
  1 small green onion
  3 tablespoons tahini
  1/2 teaspoon salt or to taste
  2 gloves garlic
  1 tablespoon Italian herbs

Place all ingredients in a blender and blend until smooth.

Avocado Salad Dressing

Avocados are used in making this favorite tasty salad dressing.

  2 medium ripe avocados
  3 tablespoons lemon juice

1/2 teaspoon sea salt, to taste
pinch of dill crushed
1/2 medium onion
1/2 cup cilantro, finely chopped
1/4 cup water

Remove skin and seed from the avocado. Then cut it into pieces and place in blender with all the other ingredients. Blend until smooth. Delicious on salad greens.

Caesar Salad Dressing

This creamy dressing is very delicious. You can add a pinch of dill if desired. This dressing goes well with any green or steamed vegetables. Stores well in the refrigerator.

1/3 cup cashew nuts
1 tablespoon tahini
1/2 cup nut milk, unsweetened
3 teaspoons garlic powder
2 tablespoons lemon juice
2 teaspoons Mrs. Dash, Italian herbs
1/2 teaspoon salt to taste

In a high-speed blender, blend cashews and milk until smooth. Then add the other ingredients until smooth

Strawberry Dressing

This dressing combines well with fresh vegetables or salad dressing. It is also delicious on waffles and pancakes and stores well in the refrigerator.

1 cup fresh strawberries, chopped

   1/3 cup dried cranberries
   1/3 cup walnuts
   1/2 cup white grape juice
   3 tablespoons lemon juice

In a high-speed blender, blend walnuts and white grape juice until smooth. Then add the other ingredients until smooth.

Orange Ginger Dressing

This dressing goes well with fresh vegetables. It can also be used in preparing stir-fry tofu. Best when used freshly made.

   2 small oranges
   1 teaspoon fresh ginger, grated
   1 tablespoon lemon
   2 tablespoons soy sauce
   1/2 cup water
   2 tablespoons tahini

In a high-speed blender, blend all the ingredients until smooth.

DESSERTS

Vegan Gluten-Free Black Bean Brownies

Easy and delicious recipe. Please watch your portion, and don't overdo it.

   2 1/2 tablespoons flaxseed meal (and 6 tablespoons water)
   1 (15-ounce) can black beans, rinsed and drained
   3 tablespoons tahini
   3/4 cup carob powder

1/4 teaspoon sea salt

1 teaspoon pure vanilla extract

1/2 cup agave

1 1/2 teaspoons baking powder

1/4 cup crushed walnuts or pecans

Preheat oven to 350 degrees Fahrenheit. Lightly grease a 12-slot standard-size muffin pan. Prepare flax eggs by combining flaxseed and water in the bowl of the food processor; pulse a couple of times and then let it rest for a few minutes. Add the remaining ingredients (except walnuts) and pulse for about 3 minutes until smooth. If the batter is too thick, add a tablespoon or two of water and pulse again. Evenly distribute the batter into the muffin tin and smooth the top with spoon. Sprinkle with crushed walnuts. Bake for 20 to 26 minutes or until the tops are dry and the edges start to pull apart. Remove from the oven and let cool for 30 minutes before removing from pan. Store in an airtight container for a few days. Refrigerate to keep longer.

Banana Peanut Butter Ice Cream

This ice cream is fat free and delicious.

3 frozen, ripe bananas, cut in pieces

2 tablespoons peanut butter

1/4 cup almond milk

With blender on ice cream or frozen-dessert mode, blend all the ingredients together until smooth; if needed, add a small amount of almond milk.

Banana Coconut Ice Cream

You can add a pinch of nutmeg or cinnamon if desired. Remember to be cautious with desserts. Do not overeat. Stores well in freezer.

> 6 frozen, ripe bananas, cut in pieces
> 1/2 (15-ounce) can coconut cream

With high-speed blender in ice cream mode, blend bananas and coconut cream until smooth.

Papaya Banana Ice Cream

This is one of my favorite desserts. It is delicious and stores well in the freezer.

> 4 cups frozen, ripe bananas, cut in pieces
> 3 cups frozen, ripe papayas, cut in pieces
> 1/2 cup almond milk
> 3 tablespoons nondairy milk powder

With a high-speed blender on ice cream or frozen-dessert mode, blend all the ingredients until smooth.

Strawberry Banana Sorbet

This simple frozen fruit dessert is great for any age. You can use any type of frozen fruit.

> 3 cups frozen strawberry, cut in pieces
> 2 cups frozen bananas, cut in pieces
> 1/2 cup fruit juice

With a high-speed blender on ice cream or frozen-dessert mode, blend all the ingredients until smooth.

Berry Sorbet

This is a great dessert to enjoy on a hot summer day. These fruits are loaded with vitamins, minerals, and antioxidants.

    2 cups frozen strawberries, cut in pieces
    1 cup frozen blueberries
    1 cup frozen blackberries
    1 cup frozen cherries
    1/2 cup white grape juice

With a high-speed blender on frozen-dessert mode, blend all the ingredients until smooth.

WHERE DO YOU GO FROM HERE?

So you are finally at the end of the book but the beginning of your journey to amazing health and longevity. It is my hope that you will use the information that you received wisely. I am sure that you will agree with me that my program is like none other you have seen before. You were probably asked to incorporate unusual foods into your diet and to make and to avoid some foods that you might love. Some of the information given might have been new and other aspects difficult to adopt. I encourage you to take small steps and reward yourself for goals achieved. Now if you fail, don't be afraid to get up and move on. Remember, success can only be gained if you get to the finish line.

It is my firm belief that education is fundamental to effect positive changes, so be prudent and wise with the information that I have laid out in this book. Allow me to reinforce that the food that you chose to enjoy could either be the number one risk factor to the illnesses that you are currently faced with or be *medicine* protecting you from chronic diseases. As mentioned in the chapter on exercise, there is a wealth of scientific research to support exercise as an essential key factor to good health, so keeping your body in motion is vital. Maintaining an active lifestyle will improve fitness and health and prevent disability; therefore, as you complete one fitness level of this program, please move on to the next.

It is no secret that good health goes far behind our mere physical dimensions, so keep your body in full balance as you incorporate other lifestyle pearls, such as the avoidance of tobacco and alcohol use. Maintaining a healthy mind and seeking spiritual renewal through daily meditation and prayer should be part of your daily routine. Remember to be kind, forgiving, and thankful and let go of anger, vengefulness, and hatred. Negative emotions will produce hypertension, anxiety, heart disease, and early death. While good health, peace, tranquility, and long life are inevitable by-products of positive emotions.

It is not possible to have optimal health without having a great relationship with family and friends, so reach out to someone today. Share the information you have gained from this book. Become a leader and empower others as you share these success strategies to amazing health and longevity. May peace be with you as you journey forward! Please find me on Facebook or send me your story at www.cooperwellnesscenter.com.

I will see you at the corner of amazing health and longevity!

BIBLIOGRAPHY

Albert, C. A., J. M. Gaziano, W. C. Willett, et al. "Nut Consumption and Decreased Risk of Sudden Cardiac Death in the Physicians Health Study." *Arch Intern Med* 162 (2002): 1382–1387.

Alexander, D. D., D. L. Weed, P. E. Miller, and M. A. Mohamed. "Red Meat and Colorectal Cancer: A Quantitative Update on the State of the Epidemiologic Science." *J Am Coll Nutr* 34, no. 6 (2015): 521–543.

Atkinson, F. S., K. Foster-Powell, and J. C. Brand-Miller. "International Tables of Glycemic Index and Glycemic Load Values." *Diabetes Care* (2008).

Aune, D., D. S. M. Chan, R. Lau, R. Vieira, and D. C. Greenwood. "Dietary Fibre, Whole Grains, and Risk of Colorectal Cancer: Systematic Review and Dose-Response Meta-Analysis of Prospective Studies." *BMJ* (2011). bmj.com.

"Benefits of Stomach Crunches." October 11, 2012. Canton Mercy, Mercy Medical Center. https://www.cantonmercy.org/blogs/healthchat/benefits-stomach-crunches.

Blackburn, G. L. "Dietary Pattern for Weight Management and Health." *Obesity Research* 511, no. 9 (2001): 217S–218S.

Blair, S. N., H. W. Kohl, R. S. Paffenbarger Jr., et al. "Physical Fitness and All-Cause Mortality: A Prospective Study of Healthy Men and Women." *JAMA* 262 (1989): 2395–2401.

Blair, S. N., Y. Cheng, and J. S. Holder. "Is Physical Activity or Physical Fitness More Important in Defining Health Benefits?" Discussion S419–20. *Med Sci Sports Exerc* 33 (2001): S379–399.

Boyle, P. "Cancer, Cigarette Smoking, and Premature Death in Europe: A Review Including the Recommendations of European Cancer

Experts Consensus Meeting, Helsinki, October 1996." *Lung Cancer* 17 (1996): 1–60.

"Chemicals in Meat Cooked at High Temperatures and Cancer Risk." National Cancer Institute. October 19, 2015. Accessed November 4, 2015. http://www.cancer.gov/about-cancer/causes-prevention/risk/diet/cooked-meats-fact-sheet.

Chisholm, A., K. McAuley, J. Mann, et al. "A Possible Protective Effect of Nut Consumption on Risk of Coronary Heart Disease: The Adventist Health Study." *Arch Intern Med* 152 (1992): 1416–1424.

"Cigarette Smoke and Adverse Health Effects: An Overview of Research." www.ncbi.nlm.nih.gov/.../articles/PMC...

Craig, W. J. "Health Effects of Vegan Diets." *American Journal of Clinical Nutrition* (2009).

Cross, A. J. *Evidence-Based Nursing* (2012).

"Cruciferous Vegetables and Cancer Prevention." June 7, 2012. Retrieved February 18, 2016. http://www.cancer.gov/about-cancer/causes-prevention/risk/diet/cruciferous-vegetables-fact-sheet.

de Munter, J. S., F. B. Hu, D. Spiegelman, M. Franz, and R. M. van Dam. "Whole Grain, Bran, and Germ Intake and Risk of Type 2 Diabetes: A Prospective Cohort Study and Systematic Review." *PLoS Med* 4 (2007): e261.

"Dietary Fibre, Whole Grains, and Risk of Colorectal Cancer: Systematic Review and Dose-Response Meta-Analysis of Prospective Studies." bn.bmj.com.

"Eating Healthy with Cruciferous Vegetables." (n.d.) http://www.whfoods.com/genpage.php?tname=btnews&dbid=126.

"Eight Reasons to Do Squat Exercises." Mercola.com. fitness.mercola.com/sites/fitness/.../darin-steen-demonstrates-the-perfect-squat.aspx.

"Exercise: 7 Benefits of Regular Physical Activity." Mayo Clinic. www.mayoclinic.org/healthy-lifestyle/fitness/in.../exercise/art-20048389.

"Fats 101." (n.d.). Retrieved February 19, 2016. http://www.heart.org/HEARTORG/HealthyLiving/FatsAndOils/Fats-101_UCM_304494_Article.jsp#.VselSJMrJE4.

Flight, I., and P. Clifton. "Cereal Grains and Legumes in the Prevention of Coronary Heart Disease and Stroke: A Review of the Literature." *European Journal of Clinical Nutrition* (2006). nature.com.

Fraser, G. E., J. Sabate, W. L. Beeson, et al. "A Possible Protective Effect of Nut Consumption on Risk of Coronary Heart Disease: The Adventist Health Study." *Arch Intern Med* 152 (1992): 1416–1424.

Haskell, W. L. et al. "Physical Activity and Public Health: Updated Recommendation for Adults from the American College of Sports Medicine and the American Heart Association." *Med Sci Sports Exerc* 39, no. 8 (2007): 1423–1434.

"Health Benefits of Physical Activity—Exercise and Fitness Center: Tips." www.medicinenet.com.

"High Fitness Levels Are Associated with a Reduced Risk of How to Do a Bulgarian Split Squat." *Shape.* www.shape.com/fitness/videos/how-do-bulgarian-split-squat.

Hu, et al. "Frequent Nut Consumption and Risk of Coronary Heart Disease in Women: Prospective Cohort Study." *British Medical Journal* 317, no. 7169 (1998): 1341–1345.

Hu, F. B., et al. "Television Watching and Other Sedentary Behaviors in Relation to Risk of Obesity and Type 2 Diabetes Mellitus in Women." *JAMA* 289 no. 14 (2003): 1785–91.

"Identifying Whole Grain Products." (n.d.). Retrieved February 19, 2016. http://wholegrainscouncil.org/whole-grains-101/identifying-whole-grain-products.

Jacobs, D. R., and L. M. Steffen. "Nutrients, Foods, and Dietary Patterns as Exposures in Research: A Framework for Food Synergy." *Am J Clin Nutr* (2003).

Jenkins, D. J. A., and C. W. C. Kendall. "Effect of Legumes as Part of a Low Glycemic Index Diet on Glycemic Control and Cardiovascular

Risk Factors in Type 2 Diabetes Mellitus: A Randomized Controlled." (2012). archinte.jamanetwork.com.

Jiang, et al. "Nut and Peanut Butter Consumption and Risk of Type 2 Diabetes in Women." *Journal of the American Medical Association* 288, no. 20 (2002): 2554–2560.

Joshi, A. D., A. Kim, J. P. Lewinge, et al. "Meat Intake, Cooking Methods, Dietary Carcinogens, and Colorectal Cancer Risk: Findings from the Colorectal Cancer Family Registry." *Cancer Med* 4, no. 6 (2015): 936–952.

Joshipura, K. J. "The Effect of Fruit and Vegetable Intake on the Risk of Coronary Heart Disease." *Annals of Internal Medicine* 134, no. 12 (2001): 1106–1114.

Kaluza, J., A. Akesson, and A. Wolk. "Long-Term Processed and Unprocessed Red Meat Consumption and Risk of Heart Failure: A Prospective Cohort Study of Women." *Int J Cardiol* 193 (2015): 42–46.

Kastorini, C. M., and D. B. Panagiotakos. "Dietary Patterns and Prevention of Type 2 Diabetes: From Research to Clinical Practice: A Systematic Review." *Current Diabetes Reviews* (2009). http://ingentaconnect.com.

Knai, C., J. Pomerleau, K. Lock, and M. McKee. "Getting Children to Eat More Fruit and Vegetables: A Systematic Review." *Preventive Medicine* (2006).

Kubzansky, L. D., and I. Kawachi. "Going to the Heart of the Matter: Do Negative Emotions Cause Coronary Heart Disease?"

"Legumes and Soybeans: Overview of Their Nutritional Profiles and Health Effects." *American Journal of Clinical Nutrition* (1999).

"Links between Processed Meat and Colorectal Cancer." World Health Organization. October 29, 2015. Accessed November 4, 2015. http://www.who.int/mediacentre/news/statements/2015/processed-meat-cancer/en/.

Lippi, G., C. Mattiuzzi, and F. Sanchis-Gomar. "Red Meat Consumption and Ischemic Heart Disease: A Systematic Literature Review." *Meat Sci* 108 (2015): 32–36.

Liu et al. "Whole-Grain Consumption and the Risk of Coronary Disease: Results from the Nurse's Health Study." *American Journal of Clinical Nutrition* 70, no. 1 (2000): 412–419.

Liu, R. H. "Health Benefits of Fruit and Vegetables Are from Additive and Synergistic Combinations of Phytochemicals." *American Journal of Clinical Nutrition* (2003).

Liu, R. H. "Potential Synergy of Phytochemicals in Cancer Prevention: Mechanism of Action." *Journal of Nutrition* (2004).

Liu, S., M. J. Stampfer, F. B. Hu, et al. "Whole-Grain Consumption and Risk of Coronary Heart Disease: Results from the Nurses' Health Study." *Am J Clin Nutr* 70 (1999): 412–419.

"Loneliness, Marriage, and Cardiovascular Health." *European Journal of Preventive Cardiology* 23 (2016): 1242–1244.

Madell, R. "Good Fats, Bad Fats, and Heart Disease." *Healthline*, 2016. http://www.healthline.com/health/heart-disease/good-fats-US.

Mancini, M., and J. Stamler. "Diet for Preventing Cardiovascular Diseases: Light from Ancel Keys, Distinguished Centenarian Scientist." *Nutr Metab Cardiovasc Dis* 14 (2004): 52–57.

"Meat Consumption and Cancer Risk." The Physicians Committee. www.pcrm.org/health.

"Meat Is Linked to Higher Cancer Risk, WHO Report Finds." *New York Times*. www.nytimes.com/.../health/report-links-some-types-of-cancer.

Mellen, P. B., T. F. Walsh, and D. M. Herrington. "Whole-Grain Intake and Cardiovascular Disease: A Meta-Analysis." *J Nutr Metab Dis* 18, no. 4 (2008): 283–290.

Mercola, J. "Stress Linked to Cancer." (2010). Mercola.com. http//www.sites/articles/archive/2010/02/04/stress-linked-to-cancer.aspx.

Messina, M. J. "Nutrition and Healthy Eating." (n.d.). Retrieved February 19, 2016. http://www.mayoclinic.org/healthy-lifestyle/nutrition-and-healthy-eating/in-depth/fat/art-20045550?pg=2.

"Nutrition and Healthy Eating." September 22, 2015. Retrieved February 18, 2016. http://www.mayoclinic.org/healthy-lifestyle/nutrition-and-healthy-eating/in-depth/fiber/art-20043983?pg=2.

Olshansky, D. J. Passaro, R. C. Hershow, et al. "A Potential Decline in Life Expectancy in the United States in the Twenty-First Century." *New England Journal of Medicine* 352 (2005): 1138–1145.

Paffenbarger, R. S. Jr., R. T. Hyde, C. C. Hsieh, et al. "Physical Activity, Other Lifestyle Patterns, Cardiovascular Disease, and Longevity." *Acta Med Scand Suppl* 711 (1986): 85–91.

"Physical Activity and Health: Physical Activity." Center for Disease Control (CDC). https://www.cdc.gov/physicalactivity/.../pa.

"Positive Emotions and Your Health." *NIH News in Health*, August 2015. https://newsinhealth.nih.gov/issue/aug2015/feature1.

Poulain, M., A. Herm, and G. Pes. "The Blue Zones: Areas of Exceptional Longevity around the World." pubs.niaaa.nih.gov/.../135-143.ht...

Rajaram, S., and J. Sabaté. "Health Benefits of a Vegetarian Diet." *Nutrition* (2000). nutritionjrnl.com.

"Red Meat Consumption: An Overview of the Risks and Benefits." https://www.meatinstitute.org/index.php?ht=a/GetDocumentAction/i/.

Rehm, J. "National Institute on Alcohol Abuse and Alcoholism." *Alcohol Research & Health* 34, no. 2.

Ricard, M., A. Lutz, and R. J. Davidson. "Mind of the Meditator." *Sci Am* 311, no. 5 (2014): 38–45.

"Risk in Red Meat?" National Institutes of Health (NIH). March 26, 2012. https://www.nih.gov/...research.../risk-red-me.

Sabate, J. "Nut Consumption, Vegetarian Diets, Ischemic Heart Disease, and All-Cause Mortality: Evidence from Epidemiologic Studies." *Am J Clin Nutr* 70 (Suppl) (1999): 5005–5035.

Sacks, et al. "Effects on Blood Pressure of Reduced Dietary Sodium and the Dietary Approach to Stop Hypertension." *New England Journal of Medicine* 344, no. 1 (2001): 3–10.

Saha, S. P. National Center for Biotechnology Information, 2007.

Schatzkin, A., T. Mouw, Y. Park, et al. "Dietary Fiber and Whole-Grain Consumption in Relation to Colorectal Cancer in the NIH-AARP Diet and Health Study." *Am J Clin Nutr* 85 (2007): 1353–1360.

Schatzkin, et al. "Dietary Fiber and Whole-Grain Consumption in Relation to Colorectal Cancer in the NIH-AARP Diet Health Study." *American Journal of Clinical Nutrition* 85, no. 5 (2007): 1353–1360.

"Seven Amazing Benefits of Walking Lunges." *StyleCraze*. August 4, 2016. www.stylecraze.com.

"Seven Science-Based Health Benefits of Drinking Enough Water." https://authoritynutrition.com/7-health-benefits-of-water/.

Slavin, J. L., and B. Lloyd. "Health Benefits of Fruits and Vegetables." *Nutrition: An International Review Journal* (2012).

"Sleep and Health: Need Sleep, Healthy Sleep." Harvard University. healthysleep.med.harvard.edu/need-sleep/whats-in-it-for.../.

"Social Relationships and Health." *Journal of Health and Social Behavior* 51, no. 1 (Suppl) (2010): S54–S66. hsb.sagepub.com/content/51/1_suppl/S54.short.

"Spirituality." University of Maryland Medical Center. umm.edu/health/medical/altmed/.../spirituality.

"Staying Active." *The Nutrition Source*. Harvard T. H. Chan School of Public Health. https://www.hsph.harvard.edu/nutritionsource.

Steinmetz, K. A., and J. D. Potter. "Vegetables, Fruit, and Cancer II. Mechanisms." *Cancer Causes & Control* (1991).

Strayer, L., D. R. Jacobs Jr., C. Schairer, A. Schatzkin, and A. Flood. "Dietary Carbohydrate, Glycemic Index, and Glycemic Load and the Risk of Colorectal Cancer in the BCDDP Cohort." *Cancer Causes Control* 18 (2007): 853–863.

Sun, Q., D. Spiegelman, R. M. van Dam, et al. "White Rice, Brown Rice, and Risk of Type 2 Diabetes in US Men and Women." *Arch Intern Med* 170 (2010): 961–969.

"Ten Things That Happen When You Do Planks Every Day." www.naturallivingideas.com/10-things-that-happen-when-you-do-planks-every-day/.

Terry, P., E. Giovannucci, and K. B. Michels. "Fruit, Vegetables, Dietary Fiber, and Risk of Colorectal Cancer." *Journal of the National Cancer Institute* (2001). jnci.oxfordjournals.org.

"The Benefits of Physical Activity for Health and Well-Being." www.c3health.org/wp.../C3-review-of-physical-activity-and-health-v-1-20110603.pd.

"The Health Benefits of Strong Relationships." Harvard Health. www.health.harvard.edu/.../the-health-benefits-of-strong-relationships.

"The Spirituality, Religion, and Health Research." www.faithandhealthconnection.org/the.../web.

"The Truth about Fats: The Good, the Bad, and in the Between." *The Family Health Guide*. Harvard Health Publication, 2015. Retrieved July 2, 2016. http://www.health-harvard.edu/stayinghealth/the-truth-about-fats-bad-and-good.

Umberson, D., and Montez, J. K. "Social Relationship and Health: A Flash Point for Health Policy." *Journal of Behavioral Science* 87, no. 6 (2010): 957–961.

Unger, R. H. "Reinventing Type 2 Diabetes: Pathogenesis, Treatment, and Prevention." *JAMA* 299 (2008): 1185–1187.

Van Duyn, M. A. S., and E. Pivonka. "Overview of the Health Benefits of Fruit and Vegetable Consumption for the Dietetics Professional: Selected Literature." *Journal of the American Dietetic Association* (2000).

Venn, B. J., and J. I. Mann. "Cereal Grains, Legumes, and Diabetes." *European Journal of Clinical Nutrition* (2004). http://nature.com.

Vienna Yearbook of Population Research 11, Special issue on Determinants of Unusual and Differential Longevity (2013): 87–108.

Wang et al. "Whole and Refined Grain Intakes and the Risk of Hypertension in Women." *American Journal of Clinical Nutrition* 86, no. 2 (2007): 472–479.

Wang, X., X. Lin, Y. Y. Ouyang, et al. "Red and Processed Meat Consumption and Mortality: Dose-Response Meta-Analysis of Prospective Cohort Studies." *Public Health Nutr* (July 6, 2015). doi: 10.1017/S1368980015002062.

"What Are the Benefits of Sunlight?" *Healthline*. www.healthline.com/health/depression/benefits-sunlight.

White, E. G. *Counsels on Health: Physical Exercise*. Hagerstown, MD: Review & Herald Publishing Association, 1870.

"Why Is Drinking Water Important?" *Medical News Today. J Psychosom Res* Apr–May 48, no. 4–5 (2000): 323–337.

"Why We Got Fatter During the Fat-Free Food Boom." (n.d.) Retrieved February 19, 2016. http://www.npr.org/sections/thesalt/2014/03/28/295332576/why-we-got-fatter-during-the-fat-free-food-boom.

World Cancer Research Fund/American Institute for Cancer Research. "Food, Nutrition, Physical Activity and the Prevention of Cancer: A Global Perspective." *American Institute of Cancer Research* (2007).

Wu, H., A. J. Flint, Q. Qi, et al. "Association between Dietary Whole Grain Intake and Risk of Mortality: Two Large Prospective Studies in US Men and Women." *JAMA Intern Med* 175, no. 3 (2015): 373–384.

Educate yourself with

the *Get Healthy with Dr. Cooper* DVD series.

Enjoy the healing power of a healthy lifestyle.
Learn simple steps toward a healthier, happier, and more abundant life.

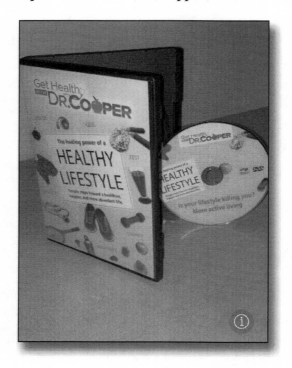

Topics

1. Is Your Lifestyle Killing You?
2. Choosing Healthy Carbohydrates and Fats
3. The Healing Power of Water / The Healing Power of Sleep
4. Maintaining Healthy Weight / Reversing Hypertension Naturally
5. Reversing Diabetes Parts 1 and 2
6. The Health Benefits of Sunshine / The Mind-Body Connection
7. Cancer Prevention / Access to Health Care Screening

Order today at www.cooperwellnesscenter.com.

Want a short, quick read on health and the Creator?

Order *My Health and the Creator* Pamphlets

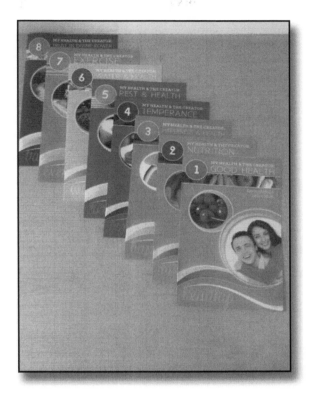

Order now at www.cooperwellnesscenter.com.

INDEX

exercise and, 54
fruits and vegetables and, 42, 43
improvement in after twelve weeks
    on program at Cooper
    Wellness Center, 116
legumes and, 38
potassium and, 41
prayer/meditation and, 106
sleep and, 81
sodium and, 49
sun and, 78
blue zone phenomenon, health facts
    about, 109–110
The Blue Zone, 42
Blueberry-Oatmeal Pancakes
    (recipe), 189
body mass index chart, 62
bowel regularity, 37, 69
brain, as wired by habitual actions, 14
bran (of grain), 22
bread (recipe), 195
breakfast recipes, 182–196
bridge (exercise), 157
brown rice
    compared to white rice, 25
    recipes, 210, 214–215
Bulgarian split squat (exercise), 165–166
burgers (recipes), 201–202, 211–
    212, 223
burpee jack (exercise), 141
burritos (recipes), 183, 211

C

Caesar Salad Dressing (recipe), 249
caffeine, 104
calcium, 32, 33, 40
calf raise (exercise), 150
calories, consumption of inappropriately
    large amounts of, 3

cancer
    anger and, 90
    colorectal cancer, risk of, 27
    effect of diet and exercise on risk
        of, xvi
    fat and, 33
    fruits and vegetables and, 39, 43
    legumes and, 35, 38
    physical exercise and, 53, 71
    polycyclic aromatic hydrocarbons
        and, 48
    preventive screening for, 92–93
    processed meat and, 47, 48, 49
    prostate cancer screening, 93
    social relationships and, 97
    sun and, 77–78
    tobacco use and, 103–104
    whole (unprocessed) grains and,
        27, 68
canned items, list of to have in pantry, 20
Cantu, Mr. (patient), 13–14
carbohydrates
    bad carbs, 25
    complex carbohydrates, 35, 36, 68
    in endosperm, 22
    good carbs, 25
cardiovascular disease
    anger and, 89
    dietary fiber and, 69
    emotions and, 87
    meats and, 48, 49
    sun and, 78
    tobacco use and, 104
    whole (unprocessed) grains and, 24
cardiovascular health
    fruits and vegetables and, 42
    sleep and, 81
Caribbean Curried Tofu (recipe),
    199–200
Cashew Brown Rice Loaf (recipe), 210

271

diabetes. *See also* type 2 diabetes
  blindness and, 4
  causes of, 3
  and coronary artery disease, 4
  diet and exercise and, xvi
  dietary fiber and, 69
  fats and, 30, 33
  fruits and vegetables and, 39–40,
    43–44
  green vegetable consumption and,
    39–40
  inactivity and, 71
  nuts and seeds and, 31
  obesity as increasing risk of, 4
  physical exercise and, 53, 54, 56
  and renal failure, 4
  sleep and, 86
  and stroke, 4
  sun and, 78
  whole (unprocessed) grains and,
    23, 24–25
Dietary Approaches to Stop Hypertension
    (DASH), 27, 43
dietary factor, as leading risk factor
    of early death (US and other
    Western countries), xvi
dietary fat, as major energy source, 29
dietary risk factor, as leading cause of
    chronic diseases and death, 47
dips (recipes), 245–246
diverticulosis, 23, 38, 69
divine intervention, seeking of, 14
double leg lift (exercise), 163
Dr. Cooper's Oats-on-the-Go (recipe),
    195–196
Dr. Cooper's Rosemary-Lemon Tofu
    Kabobs (recipe), 208–209
dried fruits, list of to have in pantry, 19

E

Easy Green Pea Soup (recipe), 240
eating late, avoidance of, 119–120
eating out, choosing wisely, 118–119
eggplant (recipe), 205, 213
Eggplant Roll-Ups (recipe), 213
Eggplant Zucchini Bake (recipe),
    213–214
eggs (recipes), 186–187, 190–191
elevated bridge (exercise), 167
emotions
  health facts about, 86–87
    negative emotions, xviii, 15, 89, 256
    positive emotions, 87, 107, 256
endosperm (of grain), 22
energy-dense diets, 3–4
enriched grains, 23
environmental factors, and risk of
    overeating, 3–4
Ephesians 4:31–32, 89
epinephrine, 81
equipment, list of to have in pantry, 20
evidence-based plans, xvi
exercise
  benefits of, 53, 54
  choice of, 55–56
  fitness levels, 124
  importance of, xvii, 11, 53
  recommended daily requirements,
    54, 71
  starting slow, 55
  US statistic, 53
exercises
  air squats, 131
  all-four kick-backs, 135
  bicep curl, 146
  bicycles, 143
  bilateral leg raise, 137
  bridge, 157

Green Smoothie (recipe), 188
Guacamole (recipe), 245

H

hamstring stretch (exercise), 147
Harvard Medical School, 43
Harvard School of Public Health, 30
HbA1c levels, 40, 57, 117
HDL (good cholesterol), 30, 31, 54
health, as a choice, not predestined, 3
health care industry, as looking to
    address current crisis, 10
health care provider, making visit
    with, 57
health goals, definition of, xviii
health status assessment, 59–61
heart disease, whole (unprocessed)
    grains and, 24
heart rate, 54, 87, 104
Heart-Healthy Bean Chili (recipe), 197
hemorrhoids, 38
hepatitis B vaccine, 93
Hepburn, Audrey, 80
herbs and spices, list of to have in pantry,
    19–20
hip abduction (exercise), 175
hip raise (exercise), 157
Hippocrates, xvii, 10, 110, 179
holistic approach, 58
hope, importance in believing in, 5
hormones, 29, 80–81, 87, 89
Hot Bulgur Wheat Cereal (recipe),
    191–192
Huevos Rancheros (recipe), 190–191
Hummus (recipe), 200–201
Hummus and Veggie Wrap (recipe), 198
the hundred (exercise), 155
hypertension
    anger and, 89
    causes of, 3, 48

diet and exercise and, xvi
fruits and vegetables and, 39
legumes and, 37
meats and, 48
negative emotions and, 15, 87, 256
obesity as increasing risk of, 4
physical exercise and, 53, 56
sleep and, 86
and whole (unprocessed) grains, 27

I

ice cream (recipes), 251–252
immature legumes, 36
immunizations, 93
inactivity
    health facts about, 71–72
    mortality and, 53
    obesity and, 71, 83
    as root cause of current health
        crisis, 10
Indian cuisine, when eating out, 119
Indian Lentil Soup (recipe), 236
Indian Rice (recipe), 216–217
influenza vaccine, 93
insulin resistance, 4, 30
intestinal discomfort, reduction of,
    37–38
iron, 21, 23, 32, 33, 36, 68
Italian cuisine, when eating out, 118
Italian Minestrone (recipe), 234
Italian White Bean Soup (recipe),
    232–233

J

Jamaican Cornmeal Porridge
    (recipe), 191
Jamaican Kidney Bean Soup (recipe),
    237–238
Jamaican Stewed Peas (recipe), 209–210

275

vegetables
blood pressure and, 42, 43
cancer and, 43
coronary artery disease and, 42
diabetes and, 39–40, 43–44
examples of, 40
as focus of health plan, 11
how and how much to consume, 41–42
hypertension and, 39, 43
obesity and, 45
recipes, 193, 206–207, 209–210, 213–214, 221–222, 224–225, 228–229, 231–236, 237–241, 243
recommended daily requirements, 39–40
stroke and, 42
Veggie Wrap with Guacamole (recipe), 221–222
vitamin A, 29, 40
vitamin B1, 99
vitamin C, 40, 41
vitamin D, 29, 77, 78
vitamin E, 23, 29, 33, 68
vitamin K, 29, 40
vitamins, 22, 24, 29, 35, 41, 42, 43, 118

W

waffles (recipes), 186, 194–195
wall push-up (exercise), 144
Walnut Balls (recipe), 224
water
benefits of, xviii
health facts about, 74–75
intake of, 10, 16, 58
weight loss
after twelve weeks on program at Cooper Wellness Center, 113

benefits of nonstarchy vegetables for, 40
eating fats as important for, 32
factors that promote, 25
physical exercise and, 54
water and, 75
White, E. G., 72
white rice, compared to brown rice, 25
whole (unprocessed) grains
and cancer, 27, 68
compared to refined (processed) grains, 21–24
dietary guidelines for, 23
examples of products with, 22
fiber content in, 26
as focus of health plan, 11
health benefits of, 23–24
and heart disease, 24
and hypertension, 27
legumes as complementary protein to, 37
protein content in, 50
recommended daily requirements, 68, 69
specialness of, 23
and type 2 diabetes, 24–25
ways to increase consumption of, 28
whole person health, xviii, 58
Whole Wheat Pancakes (recipe), 185
Wild Rice and Mushroom Pilaf (recipe), 216
Women's Health Study, 27
World Health Organization (WHO), 96
wraps (recipes), 198, 221–222

Z

zinc, 32, 33, 36
Zucchini and Cauliflower Soup (recipe), 233

Made in the USA
Middletown, DE
24 October 2020